Dr. Lani's *No-Nonsense* Bone Health Guide

Praise for *Dr. Lani's* No-Nonsense *Bone Health Guide*

"Every once in a while, a highly successful health practitioner sets aside time and energy to generously share their vast knowledge for public benefit. In her *No-Nonsense Bone Health Guide* Dr. Lani Simpson does just that, and she does it comprehensively. Whether you are interested in assessing your personal fracture risk, understanding the ins and outs of bone density testing, or learning about bone drugs, Dr. Lani is here to help you. Learn, enjoy, and build better bones—bones that will last a lifetime!"

— Susan E. Brown, PhD
Director, Center for Better Bones
Author of *Better Bones, Better Body* and *The Acid-Alkaline Food Guide*

"Balanced and fair in her approach to treatment, Dr. Simpson discusses dietary changes, exercise options, supplements, and medication. Along the way she has made the complex topic of bone metabolism approachable and relevant. An important read for providers and patients alike, or as she says, 'anyone with a skeleton.'"

— Robert Purchase, MD
Orthopedic Surgeon
Creator of the Orthopedic Patient Project

"Strong, supple bones demand more than calcium supplements. In *Dr. Lani's No-Nonsense Bone Health Guide,* this world-renowned specialist provides a comprehensive nutrition, exercise, and lifestyle plan to support and maintain healthy bones at any decade."

— JJ Virgin, CNS, CHFS
Celebrity Nutrition and Fitness Expert
New York Times bestselling author of *The Virgin Diet*

"Lani is a blessing for those of us who need guidance about complicated medical choices. I am so grateful and relieved that I can turn to her for advice about the most effective medicines, nutritional supplements, and approaches. She combines the best of traditional and complementary approaches. In short, she is a gem."

— Patricia Ellsberg
Social-Change Activist, Meditation Teacher, and Coach

"Absolutely essential reading for anyone with osteoporosis. Dr. Simpson provides a welcomed, balanced view on the pros and cons of bone mineral density (DXA) exams and the medications currently being used to treat osteoporosis. She also lays out a comprehensive map for you to follow to improve your bone health and reduce fracture risk through a natural approach using diet, supplementation, and exercise. If I were to write a sequel to my book on osteoporosis, this would be it."

— R. Keith McCormick, DC, CCSP
Author of *The Whole-Body Approach to Osteoporosis*

"Finally! An integrative doctor who has the courage to shine the light on the misconceptions about the DXA test, the diagnostic gold standard. If you've been diagnosed with osteopenia or osteoporosis, or have a family member who's been diagnosed, this is the book for you! The vast depth of bone knowledge is presented in easy-to-understand language. I've referred to Dr. Lani in the past and will continue to do so. She guides her clients to a deeper understanding with bone-saving, practical tools."

— Irma Jennings, CHC
Holistic Bone Coach
www.food4healthybones.com

"AMAZING! Dr. Lani's guide is 'all you really wanted to know about bone health but were afraid to ask.' She injects sense and wisdom into a potentially frightening medical field previously clouded with misinformation. This book is truly a MUST READ for everyone."

— Richard L. Shames, MD
Author of *Thyroid Power* and *Feeling Fat, Fuzzy, or Frazzled?*

"I have known and worked with Dr. Simpson for the past twenty years. I consider her one of the foremost experts on osteoporosis. Her approach is integrative, and her knowledge regarding bone is impressive."

— Judy Lane, NP, MS, RN, PA

"Lani and I have worked together for many years. She is a wonderful resource for topics regarding menopause and osteoporosis. She takes her time to resolve difficult cases, and her integrative approach is a breath of fresh air."

— Lisa Keller, MD, OB-GYN

"Dr. Simpson is my go-to source regarding bone health. She is the expert. She offers breadth and depth for patients who seek accurate diagnostic information regarding their bone scans and laboratory findings along with sound nutritional and exercise recommendations. She is a diligent researcher with leading-edge, relevant applications."

— Dr. Leslie Hewitt, DC
CEO, The WOW Talks
www.TheWOWTalks.com

"Dr. Simpson has done her homework and provides detailed and clearly written information that will help anyone understand and improve their bone health and quality of life. As a holistic nutritionist I appreciate her use of real foods and exercise as first-line therapy for bone maintenance. Well done!"

— Laura J. Knoff, BSc
Nutrition Consultant
Author of *The Whole-Food Guide to Overcoming Irritable Bowel Syndrome*

*For my beloved family, Audrey and Sam,
whose unwavering love, support, and patience
made this book possible.*

*Also dedicated in loving memory of
Russell, Doris, and Steve Simpson.*

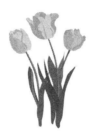

DR. LANI'S
No-Nonsense
Bone Health Guide

The Truth about Density Testing,
Osteoporosis Drugs
and Building Bone Quality
at Any Age

Lani Simpson, DC, CCD

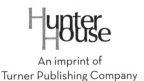

An imprint of
Turner Publishing Company

Turner Publishing Company
424 Church Street • Suite 2240 • Nashville, Tennessee 37219
445 Park Avenue • 9th Floor • New York, New York 10022
www.turnerpublishing.com

Library of Congress Cataloging-in-Publication Data
Simpson, Lani.
Dr. Lani's no-nonsense bone health guide : the truth about density testing,
osteoporosis drugs and building bone quality at any age / Lani Simpson, DC, CCD
pages cm
Includes bibliographical references and index.
isbn 978-0-89793-661-3 (pbk.) — isbn 978-0-89793-662-0 (ebook)
1. Osteoporosis. 2. Osteoporosis — Alternative treatment.
3. Bone densitometry. I. Title.
RC931.O73S55 2014
616.7'16 — dc23   2013040296

Project Credits
Cover Design: Brian Dittmar Design, Inc.
Cover Photo: Reenie Raschke   Copy Editor: Kelley Blewster
Book Production: John McKercher   Indexer: Nancy D. Peterson
Illustrations: Susan Klincsek Szecsi   Managing Editor: Alexandra Mummery
Developmental Editors: Kelley Blewster,   Publicity Coordinator: Martha Scarpati
Kirsten Enriquez, Jude Berman,   Rights Coordinator: Diane Gedymin
Mary Claire Blakeman   Publisher: Kiran S. Rana

Printed and bound by Sheridan Books, Ann Arbor, Michigan
Manufactured in the United States of America

9 8 7 6 5   First Edition   16 17 18

Contents

Foreword

Over the past twenty years, I have enjoyed a professionally collaborative and warm personal friendship with Dr. Lani Simpson. We share a mutual passion for bone health and have spent many hours discussing our clinical approaches to the treatment and care of patients with osteoporosis. While to some this may appear an unusual collaboration (Dr. Simpson is an alternative practitioner of chiropractic medicine, and I am a research-focused, academic medical doctor), over the years we have found great benefit in listening to and learning from each other. She, I believe, has become quite a good diagnostician of osteoporosis, and I have become more holistic in my approach to patient care. I am privileged to write this Foreword to her book.

Dr. Simpson has written a detailed and highly accessible guide for anyone interested in the diagnosis and care of patients with osteoporosis. It is beneficial to those wanting to prevent the disease, the newly diagnosed, and anyone interested in knowing more about this common and often debilitating condition. Her book comprehensively covers all areas of osteoporosis, including topics that few others address, for example, the quality and reliability of bone mineral density tests. In addition, she includes detailed discussions of many of the pitfalls both patients and practitioners often encounter.

I met Dr. Simpson when I was a professor of medicine and physiology and the director of the program in Osteoporosis and Bone Biology at the University of California, San Francisco. At that time, my research program was conducting some of the first clinical studies on the use of parathyroid hormone to build new bone in patients with osteoporosis. It was a very exciting time because until the development of Forteo, the only pharmaceuticals available for the treatment of osteoporosis were agents to prevent further bone loss. Already deeply interested in osteoporosis for her own personal reasons, Dr. Simpson asked to join me in my clinic to learn as much as she possibly could about the cutting-edge medical knowledge of osteoporosis to help her in her clinical practice. She was spongelike in her absorption of knowledge, and she has become an expert in understanding how to comprehensively treat the person who has an osteoporosis diagnosis.

In particular, I have been very impressed with Dr. Simpson's impeccable use of bone mineral density testing in the care of her patients. Building upon her expertise as a director of a radiologic imaging center (where she read and reported on X-rays and bone density measurements), Dr. Simpson was the first alternative doctor to become a certified clinical densitometrist. She maintains the quality of such measurement techniques and is also skilled at recognizing when it's appropriate to request the most up-to-date laboratory techniques so she can consider all the possible primary and secondary causes of osteoporosis in her patients. In her book, she illustrates these two key and fundamental aspects of her clinical care.

Dr. Simpson practices a balanced and integrative approach to osteoporosis patient care. She refers patients and consults with medical doctors when conventional medicine is needed, all the while maintaining her core treatment program, which includes nutrition, exercise, and gastrointestinal health.

It has been a delight to work with Dr. Simpson and observe her growth as a clinician and health educator. She's a Bay Area gem, and I hope her book will help anyone with a concern about osteoporosis know more in order to do more about the disease.

— Claude D. Arnaud, MD, FACE
Professor Emeritus, Medicine and Physiology
University of California, San Francisco
April 2014

Acknowledgments

I wish to thank the following people, whose expertise and support—both technical and emotional—have made this book possible. Each of you has had a significant impact on my work over the years, and I thank you deeply.

Patricia Yollin for being interested enough to write a story about my work that ended up as a feature article in the *San Francisco Chronicle* and that opened so many doors, including this book opportunity. Mary Claire Blakeman, for your heartfelt work in developing this book and securing the book contract. Kiran Rana and Hunter House for believing in and publishing this book. Dr. Leslie Hewitt, for your collaborative spirit, incredible support, and WOW talks.

Jack and Gwen Simpson, Hadas Rin, Sigrid Herr, and Jeremy Nash. Paci, Larry, and Nina Goldman, Bernie and Sadie Horowitz, Germaine Deluca, Lela DaVia. Grandma Eve, Fran, Brad and Karen Martin, Ron Martin, and the rest of the Chicago tribe. LIFE Chiropractic College West; Kendra Holloway, DC; Rae Lyn Winblad, DC; Mary Joe Hart; Irene Young; Jean Kaufman; Terri Rubinstein; Carole Goldberg; Sheryl Green; Veronica Bhonsle; Carole Johnson; Dr. Joan Steinau Lester; Redwing Keyssar, RN; Alan Cook, DC; Georgette Delvoux, DC; Paula Ross, DC; Gail Edgell; Dr. Mark Schillinger; Keith McCormick, DC. Eric, Rei, Seigo, and Kodai for being the best neighbors EVER!

Lee Glickstein, Doreen Hamilton, and Kathryn Mapes-Resnik, who gently helped me learn how to share my voice though Speaking Circles. Patrice Wynne, former owner of GAIA book store, who has been there since the beginning. Ann and Lisa for providing a respite in nature for gathering and replenishing. Christopher Titmuss and Arinna Weismann, who taught me how to be mindful and how to be with silence. Wilbur Hot Springs, where much of this book was written. To the amazing crew: I am deeply saddened by the loss of the great hotel by fire, but the memories and the land are forever!

Kirsten Enriquez, for her unwavering support and coaching, Alesia Massey for jumping in at the finish line and getting it done. Debbie Kay for added editing skills. To Kathleen Cody from the Foundation for Osteoporosis Research. Adela Lopez, Apple Williams, Bonnie Halpern, Patricia Ellsberg, Miriam Garfinkel, Maggie Hochfelder, Kate Sturla, Martin Snapp, David Rittinger, Ron Drago, Cynthia Corsi, Donna Capps. Denise Ladwig, Tina Lerner, Rainbeau, Micah McClain, Jamie Greenwood, Jill Eliason, Jack and Judy Devincenzi, Margret Carlswell, Camilla Hardmeyer, and Beverly Zoller.

Thanks to all of the wonderful researchers whose papers and presentations on bone health and osteoporosis have helped me appreciate the complexities of bone. My special thanks to the following bone experts, whose work has influenced my appreciation of the complexities of bone and for generously giving their time and expertise:

To Claude Arnaud, MD, my mentor for the past eighteen years, who allowed me to question him endlessly and who was willing to teach an eager student, my heartfelt gratitude. Elliot Schwartz, MD, and Steven Harris, MD, for consulting with me on some of my most challenging cases. Lisa Keller, MD, OB-GYN, for starting the osteoporosis journey with me in 1996, when we opened the Osteoporosis Diagnostic Center for bone density testing and consultations.

Susan Brown, PhD, for writing the first book on osteoporosis *(Better Bones, Better Body)* that helped me understand bone health from a more holistic perspective.

Judy Lane, NP, for your extraordinary diagnostic skills regarding hormone balancing for women and men, which you have shared with me over the years.

Jennifer P. Schneider, MD, PhD, for your dedicated work regarding attaining a black box warning on bisphosphonate medication labels.

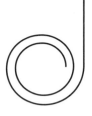

Introduction

As a chiropractor in private practice and a college-level instructor in osteology and arthrology (the study of bones and joints), I had been working with and teaching others about bone for many years when I was first diagnosed with osteoporosis at the age of forty-five.

It was 1994, and DXA (dual-energy X-ray absorptiometry) scanners were just coming on the scene as the best new technology for testing bone density. A friend of mine had a new DXA machine in his San Francisco office, so I decided to be tested, just for the experience. The scan indicated that I had osteopenia, or low bone density. I was stunned, and although I showed no reaction in my friend's office, I remember driving to my home in Berkeley, sobbing all the way. I was terrified, and this new diagnosis made me feel as if I was physically weak.

I knew that my diet was good and that I had a robust exercise program. I was physically strong and had never broken a bone. So why did I have low bone density? Something didn't seem right. That same week I obtained another bone density test at the University of California, San Francisco. This time the results were worse! My bone density read as 10 percent lower than it had been a week earlier, and *the new test results placed me in the osteoporosis category.*

I was now labeled by at least one DXA center as having a disease that I associated with old age. Furthermore, I didn't really know how serious my condition was. What did this mean on a practical level?

Did I have to stop engaging in the sports I loved, including tennis, biking, running, and roller skating? In addition, I had been told, and many of my colleagues believed, that DXA testing was the gold standard for bone density measurement. Yet it was evident from the fact that my own two tests registered scores that differed by 10 percent that the procedure could be quite inaccurate.

It was then that I decided to learn everything I could about osteoporosis—and DXA testing. Things just weren't adding up, and I knew that my bone health depended on my gaining a much deeper understanding of what healthy bone actually entailed.

One of the main reasons I wrote this book was to share my discoveries with you, because through my own journey I learned the following important lesson: *Most doctors' assessment and treatment of osteoporosis are woefully inadequate.* Therefore, anyone who wants to maintain and/or improve their bone health needs information and a perspective that are quite different from what is commonly conveyed in doctors' offices. For example:

o *Bone density testing errors are extremely common.* As a bone-health consultant who works with both patients and doctors from all over the country, I see these testing errors over and over. They often lead to inaccurate reports of bone loss (or gain), which in turn can lead to improper or unneeded treatment.

o *Most testing errors occur because of human error,* including, for example, inaccurate comparisons of initial and follow-up tests; inaccurate selection of the area of the body to be tested; improper patient positioning; and inaccurate reporting by the interpreting physician.

o *Not all states require bone density technicians to be trained in densitometry, and **no** states require this training of the doctors who interpret the test results.* (Densitometry, stated simply, is the measurement of bone density.) It is this lack of professional training that accounts for the vast majority of testing errors. The failure to require densitometry training for doctors is especially problematic. If the doctors responsible for interpreting bone density tests were trained, they could catch and correct the errors made by the test technicians.

o *Nutrition and gastrointestinal health are essentially omitted from most osteoporosis treatment plans.* Most conventional doctors do not have training in nutrition; therefore, they tend to ignore nutritional status and gastrointestinal health when it comes to assessment and treatment. But these factors are *crucial* to bone health, and many patients' bone-health problems could resolve if they were addressed.

o *Osteoporosis medications tend to be overrated and overprescribed.* Sadly, I see doctors prescribe medications for patients whose only risk for fractures is a diagnosis of osteopenia (low bone mass), or borderline osteoporosis. I see doctors prescribe medications before ordering the lab tests that could rule out secondary causes of osteoporosis. And I see doctors leave their patients on osteoporosis medications for years and years, despite the fact that long-term use of some of them is linked to an increased risk for fractures.

Make no mistake: My intention is not to undermine the value of DXA testing or osteoporosis medications. My intentions are (1) to give my readers information that will enable them to get more accurate test results, and (2) to outline a more integrative treatment option than medications alone.

For patients who have significant osteoporosis and who are at a high risk for fractures, medications can be invaluable in reducing that fracture risk. And I'm a huge believer in DXA testing—when it is done correctly, and by providers who have a solid foundation in densitometry, which you will learn about in Chapters 2 and 3. Therefore my intention is to shine a light on the problems associated with bone density testing so that this tool can be used in the most effective way possible for diagnosis.

If you have risk factors and haven't had a DXA test, my hope is that this book will motivate you to get one, because at the very least your first DXA test gives you a measure of one very important piece of information about your overall bone health. Osteoporosis is linked to a host of risk factors that cause people to lose bone long before they reach old age. Early bone-health assessments that include nutritional and gastrointestinal assessment, BMD testing, lab tests, and

evaluation of symptoms and lifestyle will go a long way toward helping you to prevent fractures.

I Don't Have Osteoporosis—
Do I Need This Book?

Yes. This book is for anyone with a skeleton. Sorry, I'm being a bit
facetious! But I really want you to understand that this book is *not*
just for people with osteoporosis, and it's *not* just for readers who are
elderly or reaching the end of middle age. This is a book for people of
all ages, because the lifestyle choices we make throughout our lives
have a direct impact on how healthy our bones will be when we're
older—and also because it's much easier to prevent osteoporosis than
to reverse it.

We usually think of osteoporosis as a disease of the elderly, but
in fact the condition often brews in the background long before it's
finally discovered. This is because, in many cases, osteoporosis develops from a failure to acquire sufficient bone mass when we're younger
and/or because of lifestyle choices or secondary conditions that cause
bone loss. Poor nutrition in childhood and adolescence, for example,
means that you won't build the bone reserves you need by the time
your body's bone-building processes slow down.

As another example, alcohol dependence, digestive problems,
hormone imbalances, and even some medications can result in bone
loss that might lead to osteoporosis. Lifestyle factors are such key
players that you can actually prevent osteoporosis if you choose a
lifestyle that gets you the nutrients and exercise you need to support
your bones. And prevention is a very good strategy, because once we
reach middle age many of us will lose bone faster than we're able to
build new bone. It becomes much more difficult to build new bone
as we get older.

This book, then, is for anyone, young or old, who wants to build
and maintain the health of their bones. If you have osteoporosis, this
book will help you to improve your bone health, and if your bones
are currently healthy, this book can help you to prevent the disease.

How to Use This Book

Although I've structured this book so that it can be read from cover to cover, some of you will find some chapters more or less relevant, depending on your situation.

In my opinion, everyone should review Chapter 4, which describes the many risk factors associated with osteoporosis. Some of them—age, height, and skeletal frame size, for example—cannot be changed. However, a great number of them *can* be addressed, and if you reduce your bone-health risk factors, your bones benefit. Understanding osteoporosis-related risk factors can also help you make treatment decisions.

Chapters 8 through 11 are also almost universally applicable. Chapter 8 addresses the importance of hormonal balance, and Chapters 9, 10, and 11 address the core requirements of any effective bone-health program: a gastrointestinal system that optimally absorbs nutrients; proper nutrition; and bone-building exercise. Whether you're trying to treat osteoporosis or trying to prevent it, GI health and a healthy, bone-building lifestyle are key. These chapters provide crucial information you may not hear from your doctor, because the Western medical model is a bit anemic and out of shape when it comes to a genuine focus on nutrition and exercise. And just as our bones depend on the right nutrients in the right amounts, so, too, do they depend on the hormones our bodies produce, which must be available in the right proportions. For some, hormone supplementation can stop bone loss.

If you've already had a BMD test, Chapters 2 and 3 can help you to understand some of the significant factors that may have impacted and even skewed your test results. If you haven't been tested yet, these chapters will guide you in asking the questions you need to ask to be sure that your tests are as accurate as they can be.

What if your doctor has told you that your bone health leaves something to be desired? Has she/he taken the time to figure out *why* this is the case? Too many doctors prescribe unnecessary medications based solely on BMD test results, but osteoporosis can arise from a host of secondary conditions, and if we can treat them, we can improve our bones. Chapter 5 shows you how to test for these conditions, and also highlights the importance of health assessments that show whether you're currently losing bone. If your doctor has recommended osteoporosis medications, Chapter 6 provides important information that can help you make a decision as to whether or when to include them as part of your treatment regimen. The most popular osteoporosis medications have serious side effects, so it's best to be sure you need them before accepting a prescription.

Finally, whether medications are appropriate for you or not, everyone should be aware of treatment alternatives. Chapter 7 lists alternative treatments that can help improve bone health. It also illuminates a key perspective that's often overlooked in the alternative-medicine world, namely, the fact that low bone density is not easily reversed, and there are no quick fixes when it comes to osteoporosis.

My hope is that this book provides those who read it with a new way of thinking about bone health. Osteoporosis is not a simple disease with simple answers. If you've been diagnosed with osteoporosis, question the diagnosis and question your doctor's recommendations for treating it. At the same time, however, know that it is not my intention that you use this book as a self-diagnostic tool. Instead, seek the expertise of qualified providers who truly understand bone health and bone density testing—and use the information in this book to guide you as you evaluate the information your providers give you.

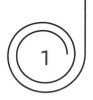

Fractures:
Facts and Fears

Unless you break one, you probably don't spend much time thinking about your bones.

If you do imagine what your skeletal structure looks like, you may envision it as a collection of dry, stiff bones, like something found in the desert. In fact, our bones are far from dried up and static. They are living tissues teeming with minerals and other nutrients.

Like we do with most invisible body parts, however, we tend to take our bones for granted—until something goes wrong with them. Whether we break a leg or get unsettling results from a bone density test, it can come as a shock if we learn that the bones we depend on to hold us up seem to be letting us down.

In my practice I regularly get calls from people concerned about the condition of their bones and their bodies. Some of these folks have sustained fractures, while others are upset, confused, or skeptical because their doctors have diagnosed them with osteoporosis or told them they're at risk for breaking their bones. Regardless of whether their fracture risk is high or low, they nevertheless feel fearful that their bodies could easily crumble beneath them.

Since many of the people I hear from are middle-aged and older adults, their fear of fractures is often tied to the fear of losing physical independence in later life. No one wants to end up immobilized in a care facility because they've broken a hip. That possibility—or worse—is borne out by statistics telling us that among hip fracture patients over the age of fifty, an estimated 40 percent will require nursing home care, and an average of 24 percent will die in the year following their fracture. It is important to note, however, that those who die following a hip fracture tend to be people who were frail before the fracture or who have other serious health problems. Nevertheless, it is disconcerting when friends or family members tell us stories of a grandmother, an uncle, or a coworker whose life went downhill after they fractured a hip.

To calm their anxieties, I first let my patients know that their fracture risk may or may not be serious, depending on their health status. Every case of osteoporosis is unique. Furthermore, few people realize that osteoporosis is a disease with gradations ranging from borderline to severe, much like cancer, which varies greatly between stage 1 and stage 4. While no one should dismiss the seriousness of osteoporosis as a disease that predisposes a person to fractures, it is also true that great numbers of people can live with the condition without ever breaking a bone, depending on their specific diagnoses, health histories, and risk factors.

It is crucial, then, to keep the statistics and stories about bone problems in perspective. This chapter is designed to help give you that perspective, along with a basic understanding of bone development and fracture types. This knowledge, coupled with the assessment tools you'll read about in forthcoming chapters, will provide you with the insight into your bone health that can help you make decisions about nutrition, exercise, supplements, potential treatments, and other factors.

Let's begin by looking at bone development.

Know How Your Bones Grow

Just prior to birth, a child's skeleton begins to transform from soft cartilage into bone, a process that continues throughout adolescence and into early adulthood. Though infants begin life with approximately 300 bones, many of them fuse together, and by adulthood the skeleton typically has only 206 bones.

Although your genes have a major impact on how fast and how well your bones develop, the process is also affected by your intake of calcium, magnesium, vitamin D, and other nutrients, as well as by your level of exercise and your exposure to stress and harmful substances in the environment. As stated earlier, your bones are comprised of dynamic living tissue with a rich blood supply, and they function, in part, as a reservoir of nutrients, primarily calcium. If you are not getting enough calcium in your diet, your bone tissue will release it into the bloodstream, thus potentially depleting the bones' reserves of this essential nutrient.

Externally, changes in the skeleton are exhibited by a child's growth, which usually hits its highest point in late adolescence. What we cannot see is the internal process of ongoing bone maintenance, in which the body remodels the skeletal structure approximately every seven to ten years throughout the life span.

For most people, bone development follows an arc that rises slowly during childhood, peaks in the late teen years, and then begins sloping downward after age thirty-five. Here is how the life cycle of bone proceeds, statistically speaking:

o Approximately 80 percent of our lifetime bone mass develops before the age of eighteen. Our bones experience their biggest growth spurt during puberty.

o Peak bone mass is achieved between the ages of twenty-five and thirty.

o After age fifty it is common to see a 0.5 to 1 percent bone loss each year in some individuals.

o Postmenopausal women can record a 1 to 3 percent annual bone loss for five to ten years after menopause, mostly attributable to declining estrogen levels. This increased bone loss can begin during the premenopausal years.

o Approximately five to ten years postmenopause, 0.5 to 1 percent annual bone loss will resume in many women. This is referred to as age-related loss.

o Men tend to follow the same patterns of bone loss as women, but ten years later.

Note: The statistics above are "facts." However, keep in mind that there are things you can do to minimize age-related bone loss.

Figure 1.1 on the next page graphically illustrates this progression.

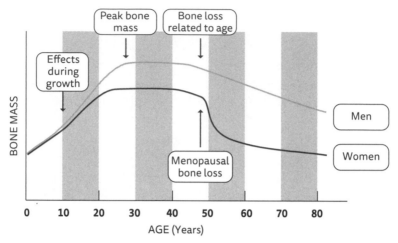

FIGURE 1.1. Age-related bone growth and loss for males and females
Source: Adapted from http://pmj.bmj.com/content/78/926/727/F2.large.jpg

What Happens When Bone Loss Occurs

As we age, fat accumulates in the bone marrow space. According to one study, "The predominant feature of age-related bone loss is the accumulation of bone marrow fat at the expense of osteoblasto-genesis [the production of new bone cells].... This accumulation of marrow fat appears to be an active process independent of estrogen since it is evident during the third and fourth decade of life [that] stem cells go [convert] to fat rather than bone."

Some people think that the aging process inevitably involves shrinking in height or fracturing bones. That assumption, however, can lead them to underestimate the importance of preventing bone loss and breaks, which could be symptoms of osteoporosis or other disease processes at work in the body. Those who adopt the attitude, "I'm just getting old" often avoid having a bone density test or taking other steps that could improve their long-term bone health. It is true that more effort is required to build and maintain bone health after your early to mid-thirties, but doing so is well worth the effort. I do not necessarily consider age-related bone loss to be "normal," and the term "age-related" can cause people to see these changes as inevitable.

Quite often, "normal" age-related loss may result from not exercising and/or from a diet that does not support bone health.

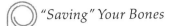 *"Saving" Your Bones*

The amount of bone you develop before age eighteen is often likened to a savings account into which you've "deposited" a bone supply that you can tap into throughout your lifetime. The biological process is more complicated than that, but essentially you start contributing to your bone "savings account" while still in the womb, and you continue making "deposits" throughout childhood and young adulthood, until reaching peak bone mass, sometime between ages twenty-five and thirty. After that, between ages thirty and thirty-five, many people, especially women, begin making "withdrawals." If you have a very small frame, smoked as a teenager, or ate a calcium-poor diet, you may have fewer reserves to draw upon for handling potential age-related or postmenopausal bone loss—and that can lead to fractures and other problems in later years. A small number of individuals may have inherited the type of genes that seem to let them get away with somewhat unhealthy lifestyles for a while before it impacts their bodies. But for nearly all of us, it is crucial to follow a diet and exercise program that helps us maintain bone health throughout our lifetimes.

Remodeling: Building Bones... or Breaking Them Down?

Like a never-ending New Year's celebration, your bones undergo a process of throwing out the old and welcoming the new right below the surface of your skin and muscles. This process—called "bone remodeling"—is a continuous cycle that recurs throughout your lifetime. It is designed to keep your skeletal structure healthy and supple by getting rid of old bone and laying down new bone. As we age, the remodeling becomes less effective, so that by the time we are in our eighties and nineties our bone is more brittle. It is possible, however, to slow down this particular aging process by eating healthy food and exercising.

Bone remodeling primarily depends on the work of two types of bone cells: osteoclasts and osteoblasts. The job of osteoclasts is to remove old bone (through a process called resorption), and the job of osteoblasts is to lay down new bone (see Figure 1.2).

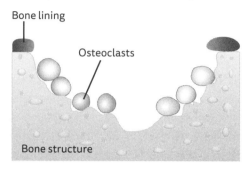

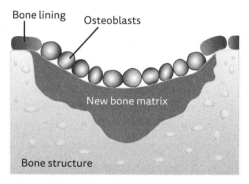

FIGURE 1.2. Bone remodeling

Here is a simple way to remember which type of bone cell does what:

○ OsteoClasts—Chew up

○ OsteoBlasts—Build up

When the body and bones are healthy, osteoclasts and osteoblasts maintain a state of equilibrium in which, starting in childhood, old bone is replaced by new bone in a steady cycle. As discussed earlier, however, that cycle changes as we grow older. After the age of thirty to thirty-five, the tendency in many people is for the osteoclasts to slowly outpace the osteoblasts' ability to lay down new bone. This is referred to as age-related bone loss and it affects nearly everyone by the age of seventy. In women, bone loss accelerates markedly as estrogen declines around the time of menopause. That's because one function of estrogen is to keep osteoclasts in check.

Osteoporosis can result from normal age-related bone loss as osteoclasts get the upper hand over osteoblasts. But osteoporosis can also arise from numerous other health issues that are not directly connected to age-related bone loss, such as anorexia, prolonged use of steroids, alcohol abuse, or hyperparathyroidism. These health issues are referred to as "secondary causes" of osteoporosis, and you'll read more about them in Chapter 5.

Much of the medical approach to treating osteoporosis is based on the idea of preventing bone loss by stopping the osteoclasts from removing old bone. Medications can effectively accomplish this goal—but long-term use of some medications actually increases fracture risk in some individuals and thus appears to compromise bone quality. You will learn more about this phenomenon in Chapter 6.

BMD: "Bone Mineral Density" Defined

One term you will encounter often in this book—and one that you need to know when it comes to understanding fracture risks and osteoporosis—is "bone mineral density" or "BMD." It refers to the concentration of minerals (such as calcium) and other materials within a bone or section of bone. Bone mineral density measurement is one of the most important tools for predicting future fracture risk: The lower the density, the higher the risk. Though it accounts for only one aspect of overall bone strength, there is a positive correlation between BMD and the mechanical strength of bones.

Mainstream medicine considers BMD a reliable benchmark of bone health, but some critics find it a less than ideal yardstick. While researchers and health care professionals may argue the point, the main thing for you to remember is that your BMD level, when accurately measured, gives you one major piece of information about the state of your bones and the possibility that they could fracture—*but it is only one piece of the whole puzzle.*

Dr. Susan Ott, a professor of medicine at the University of Washington, underscores the idea that BMD should be considered as only one among many factors that affect fracture risk. As she states, "Age, heredity, body weight, diseases, lifestyle, frailty, and amount of trauma all play important roles. The risk of a fracture due to osteoporosis can be estimated using these factors in addition to the bone density."

Note: The terms "bone density," "bone mineral density" (BMD), and "bone mass" are often used interchangeably. Technically, bone density and bone mass are not exactly the same thing—"bone mass" refers to the totality of the bone tissue while "bone density" refers only to the mineral content of bone.

Understanding Osteoporosis

The simplest way to understand the term "osteoporosis" is to break the word down into its Greek and Latin roots:

osteo = bone

porous = void spaces

osis = condition of

"Osteoporosis," then, means "porous bones." You can see the difference between this type of bone and normal bone in Figure 1.3.

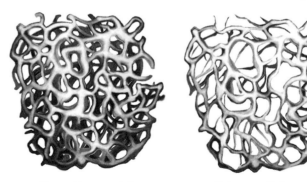

Normal bone matrix   Osteoporotic bone

FIGURE 1.3. Normal bone compared to bone with osteoporosis. The osteoporotic bone has lost some of its microarchitecture (trabeculae), thus weakening its infrastructure.

In addition, the National Institutes of Health (NIH) offers two other definitions of osteoporosis that will help expand your understanding of it:

1. "[Osteoporosis] is characterized by too little bone formation, excessive bone loss, or a combination of both."

This definition not only describes osteoporosis in terms of bone loss; it also explains how a person could be diagnosed with osteoporosis because they never built up a good bone "bank account" by the time they reached peak bone mass in their late twenties.

2. "Osteoporosis is a skeletal disorder characterized by compromised bone strength predisposing one to an increased risk of fracture. Bone strength reflects the integration of two main features: bone density and bone quality."

This definition recognizes the concepts of both bone *density* and bone *quality*. It is important to note that bone density is only one aspect of bone health (and you will see an expanded explanation of bone mineral density below). If bone density is seriously low, it is easy to imagine that both bone strength and bone quality will be compromised. However, if bone density is only somewhat low, an individual's overall bone strength may not be significantly impaired. A simple example of the importance of bone strength can be seen in the case where two people have the exact same bone mineral density measurement—but one person may be fracturing easily while the other is not. What's the difference? One answer to that question could be a difference in bone *quality*. Currently it is not possible to quantify bone quality in the same way that we can measure bone mineral density through DXA tests (see Chapters 2 and 3). But a few factors that can independently affect bone quality include smoking, poor diet, and malabsorption syndromes (which you will learn more about in Chapters 9 and 10).

Whereas the NIH describes osteoporosis as above, the World Health Organization defines osteoporosis in terms of bone density testing measurements, which are explained in greater detail in Chapter 3.

Types of Osteoporosis

Now that you've gotten a basic overview of bone development and osteoporosis, let's break down a few more of the terms and concepts you need to understand when it comes to your own bone health. Don't worry about remembering all of the details; just use this section as a helpful reference.

As with other medical conditions, different terms are used to describe the various forms of osteoporosis. Generally speaking, however, osteoporosis is classified in terms of three diagnostic categories—primary, secondary, and idiopathic:

1. *Primary osteoporosis*—includes type 1 and type 2, both of which are far more common in women than in men:
   • Type 1 results from postmenopausal estrogen loss.
   • Type 2 is caused by age-related bone loss.

2. *Secondary osteoporosis*—can be caused by a wide range of diseases, conditions, and medications. Causes include thyroid or kidney disorders; intestinal absorption problems; vitamin D deficiency; poor diet and sedentary lifestyle; and the use of various medications, including corticosteroids, proton pump inhibitors, and aromatase inhibitors (estrogen blockers), among others.

3. *Idiopathic osteoporosis*—attributed to unknown causes. In both children and adults, osteoporosis can occur in the absence of any discernible cause. For example, a rare condition called idiopathic juvenile osteoporosis can affect children; however, young patients may be able to recover lost bone. In some cases of adult osteoporosis, when no known cause has been determined through extensive lab work, the osteoporosis may be described as idiopathic. Patients requiring extensive lab work are typically those with advanced cases of osteoporosis, not borderline.

Risk Factors for Osteoporosis

Osteoporosis has a number of specific risk factors, including those shown in Table 1.1 below. Please note that this list, which was adapted from information provided by the National Institutes of Health, is only partial. Osteoporosis can also arise from a number of secondary causes, which underscores how important it is for a doctor to assess your case individually. Later, in Chapter 4, you'll find a more comprehensive discussion of risks, and you'll also learn about the pros and cons concerning the use of fracture risk calculators to evaluate your individual fracture risk.

Table 1.1. Risk Factors for Osteoporosis

Risk Factors You Cannot Change	Other Risk Factors
Gender: Women get osteoporosis more often than men	**Sex hormones:** In women: Low estrogen levels due to missing menstrual periods or menopause. In men: Low testosterone
Age: The older you are, the greater your risk	Anorexia nervosa
Body size: Small, thin women are at greater risk	**Low calcium and vitamin D intake**
Ethnicity: White and Asian women are at highest risk; African American and Latina women have a lower risk	**Medication use:** Some medicines increase risk
Family history: Osteoporosis tends to run in families	**Activity level:** Lack of exercise or long-term bed rest can cause weak bones; smoking cigarettes; drinking alcohol

Source: National Institutes of Health

How Bones Break: Basic Types of Fractures

In medical terms, a fracture is, essentially, a broken bone. To diagnose and treat fractures, however, physicians need more specific information about how and why a bone has broken, so they classify various types of breaks into different categories. You may be familiar with stress fractures, for instance. They can affect anyone but are especially seen in athletes, dancers, runners, and even soldiers—that is, in individuals whose activities cause repeated stress to certain body parts (such as the foot). This stress, in turn, can lead to fractures.

While there are numerous ways to categorize fractures, for simplicity's sake, when we are considering osteoporosis, we are interested in differentiating between two major types:

1. trauma fractures

2. osteoporosis-related fractures

The rest of this section discusses these two fracture categories, as well as compression fractures—a common type of fracture that can be attributed to trauma, osteoporosis, or a combination of both. For a graphic summary of issues that affect bone strength and fracture potential, see Figure 1.4. These various topics will be discussed in chapters to come.

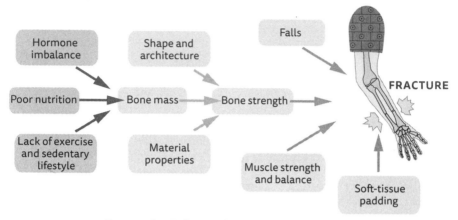

FIGURE 1.4. Factors that influence bone strength and fracture potential

Trauma Fractures

Trauma fractures result from the direct, physical impact of an event such as tumbling off a ladder, falling hard on cement, being injured in a car accident, or getting hit during a football game or other sports contest. Trauma fractures—unlike osteoporosis-related fractures—are not generally associated with an underlying weakness in the bones. Rather, they occur because the bones cannot withstand the amount of force exerted on them by the trauma event. It is important for patients who have broken a bone to determine whether or not their fracture is a trauma fracture—because even a trauma fracture could be due in part to osteoporosis or some other bone disease that has weakened the skeleton.

Of course there are gray areas. Osteoporosis may predispose some individuals to fracture a bone with less trauma than would be expected. That's why it is important to tease out the details of any activities or life events that result in a fracture, as this information can influence medical decisions.

Stress fractures are generally classified in the trauma category, because the repetitive pounding of an activity like running causes the physical stress necessary to produce hairline breaks over time. But a stress fracture can also be a red flag for low bone density or osteoporosis. It's one thing if a stress fracture occurs in a person who trains for and runs a marathon, but there could be other problems if it happens after a long walk. Stress fractures are not always visible on X-rays; an MRI or CT scan may be required to confirm them. (You may want to seek this type of assessment if it seems the area in question has not healed after four to six weeks.) If you or someone in your life experiences repeated stress fractures (or a fracture that seems to be of questionable origin), consider getting an accurate bone density test to investigate the problem further.

Note: "Insufficiency fracture" is a term you may see in medical reports. Sometimes referred to as a subtype of stress fracture, it can happen without any trauma whatsoever. Medscape explains that these fractures occur due to loss of trabeculae (see Figure 1.3 on page 14) and that they are "caused by normal or physiologic stress upon weakened bone." In other words, the bone is so weak it can collapse due to the mere stress of body weight. Insufficiency fractures are seen only in extreme cases of osteoporosis or some other bone pathology; they have also been noted in patients who have used certain osteoporosis medications for long periods.

Osteoporosis-Related Fractures

Different terms are used to identify fractures caused by or related to osteoporosis—which can be confusing when you're talking to your doctor or doing online research. The following is a list of some of the names for osteoporosis-related fractures (note that all of these terms basically mean the same thing):

o fragility fracture

o minimal- or low-trauma fracture

o low-impact fracture

o osteoporotic fracture

The World Health Organization describes all osteoporosis-related fractures as "fracture[s] caused by injury that would be insufficient to fracture a normal bone." So although the above labels differ, they all describe the types of bone breaks that occur under the conditions that define an osteoporosis-related fracture. In other words, these fractures occur:

o with minimal or no trauma

o from a standing height or lower

This means if you have osteoporosis you can fracture a bone if you trip and fall onto the floor or the street. That's a fall from a standing height, and when there is no underlying pathology, most people can fall that far without breaking a bone—although certainly there are instances when falling from a standing height can have significant impact. For instance, if someone falls hard from a standing height and breaks their wrist, it does not necessarily mean their bones are significantly weak. In advanced osteoporosis, more commonly seen in elderly patients, fractures can be caused simply by sneezing or bumping into a chair—that is, with barely any trauma.

When my older patients are unclear about whether a recent fracture could be due to osteoporosis, I sometimes ask them, "If this had happened when you were twenty-five years old, do you think you would have fractured?" Answering "no" to that question is one indication that their fractures may not be due to a specific trauma event and that further investigation is needed.

Pathologic Fractures

Osteoporosis-related fractures are actually part of a larger category of fractures that are referred to as "pathologic." As the name suggests, pathologic fractures result from pathology (i.e., from an underlying disease condition). Bone cancers, tumors, and infections, as well as osteomalacia and rheumatoid arthritis, are among the conditions that can result in bone loss and pathologic fractures. Nontraumatic fractures should always be investigated to make sure there is not an underlying pathology. This is especially true regarding fractures of the spine, where metastasis from bone cancer, for example, can result in a nontraumatic fracture.

Compression Fractures

Both osteoporosis and trauma contribute to another category of fractures that is important to know about: compression fractures. The vast majority of compression fractures affect the spine, although they can occur in other parts of the body. Compression fractures of the spine may also be described as "vertebral fractures." The most common cause of vertebral compression fractures is osteoporosis, but they can also be caused by other conditions such as those mentioned in the preceding box, "Pathologic Fractures."

The twenty-four bones that make up the spinal column, called "vertebrae," rest one on top of the other like a stack of boxes (see Figure 1.5). With a compression fracture, typically, the front (body) of the vertebra collapses to a small or large degree, possibly causing

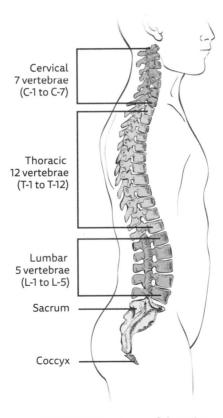

Cervical
7 vertebrae
(C-1 to C-7)

Thoracic
12 vertebrae
(T-1 to T-12)

Lumbar
5 vertebrae
(L-1 to L-5)

Sacrum

Coccyx

FIGURE 1.5. Anatomy of the spine

pain and loss of height (see Figure 1.6). Compression fractures of the spine occur most commonly in the thoracic (middle back) and lumbar (lower back) regions.

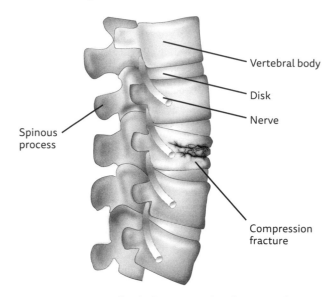

Vertebral body

Disk

Nerve

Spinous process

Compression fracture

FIGURE 1.6. Grade 2 compression fracture of one vertebra of the lumbar spine

One of the methods used to measure the extent of a compression fracture is Genant's grading system, which indicates what percentage of bone has collapsed. It classifies compression fractures as follows:

o Grade 1 (mild)—20–25 percent bone collapse

o Grade 2 (moderate)—25–40 percent bone collapse

o Grade 3 (severe)—40+ percent bone collapse

Small compression fractures do not always produce pain or much discomfort, and some people remain unaware that they have sustained a fracture. They are often discovered incidentally, when an X-ray of the spine is taken for another reason. Fractures seen on X-rays may have occurred in childhood, and sometimes it is hard for a radiologist to confirm if the fracture is relatively new or old. Multiple compression fractures can lead to the hunched-over posture seen in older adults, an image that is most commonly associated with osteoporosis. However, one, two, or even three mild compression fractures do not necessarily result in obvious disfigurement. An extremely hunched-over posture (Dowager's hump) is primarily seen in very advanced cases of osteoporosis in elderly people.

When a patient sustains a compression fracture of one or more vertebrae, a doctor may offer him or her the option of undergoing vertebroplasty or kyphoplasty. Each of these procedures presents its own problems and side effects; however, sometimes they are necessary, as a severe compression fracture can place pressure on a spinal nerve or on the spinal cord, resulting in serious pain. Though the two procedures are slightly different, they both involve inserting liquid plastic cement into the vertebral body. One procedure (kyphoplasty) involves inserting a balloon first and then injecting the cement; this procedure seems to have the best track record because the cement tends to remain where it was injected. After the procedure or even years later, complications can arise because natural bone is not as hard as plastic cement. The harder cement can make adjacent vertebrae more vulnerable to fracture due to its unforgiving nature. Down the road, researchers may develop a more flexible material, but for now, if you're considering one of these procedures, make sure to discuss your options carefully with your doctor.

Fracture FAQs

It is undeniably true that your chances of fracturing a bone depend on the specifics of your individual health profile. At the same time, bone fractures and osteoporosis present a significant public health problem to the United States population at large. But how big is that problem? And is it a problem for you? This section sheds light on those questions.

What Breaks a Bone?

Most of us have seen what happens to an overloaded supermarket paper bag when the weight of the groceries puts more pressure on the bottom of the bag than it can handle. Similarly, when a bone is hit with excess force or more pressure than it can withstand, it breaks—and this is the process that is typical of most trauma fractures that result from events like a car crash or a fall off a ladder. You can see, then, why osteoporosis fractures are sometimes referred to as "minimal trauma fractures," or "fragility fractures"—because the bones break under the minimal pressure caused by ordinary activities like stepping off a curb or even coughing. As mentioned earlier in the chapter, these types of fractures typically occur with advanced osteoporosis.

Do Fractures Have a Timeline?

Osteoporosis fractures can occur anywhere in the body. Bone density testing, which is used to diagnose osteoporosis, focuses on the following three areas of the body:

1. forearm
2. lumbar spine (lower back)
3. hip

Interestingly, fractures in these three regions seem to follow a pattern over time.

For women:

o Forearm fractures begin to increase around age forty-five to fifty and level off around age sixty-five.

o Vertebral (spine) fractures begin to increase around age fifty-five or sixty and rise linearly in frequency thereafter.

o Hip fractures increase at age sixty-five and increase exponentially thereafter.

For men:

o While forearm fractures show no increase, the incidence of lumbar spine and hip fractures rises about five to ten years later than in women.

o One quarter of all hip fractures occur in men.

o Rib fractures are more frequent in men over age thirty-five. Although men often sustain a rib fracture while playing a sport, it may be an early sign of osteoporosis that warrants further investigation, especially if the fracture was low-trauma.

These age-related patterns in the occurrence of osteoporosis fractures are due to differences in the two types of bone that make up the skeleton: cortical and cancellous (also referred to as spongy bone).

Cortical bone is the dense outer covering in which our bones are encased. Cancellous bone resembles layers of latticework that provide the inner scaffolding that makes bones light and strong. The spine and wrist are mostly made up of cancellous bone, and the hip is a mix of both types.

As we age, our cortical and cancellous bone declines at different rates. We lose cancellous bone first. Women, especially, can lose significant amounts of cancellous bone during their postmenopausal years. When osteoporosis-related fractures accelerate in the fifth and sixth decades of life, loss occurs mainly in those areas comprised primarily of cancellous bone, such as the spine and wrist.

Wrist and Hip Fractures

A wrist fracture can be one of the first signs that a postmenopausal woman has osteoporosis. A wrist fracture can also indicate a higher risk of fractures at other sites in the body. If you experience such a fracture, it is important to have your bone mineral density tested and to have your personal risk factors assessed (see Chapter 5). Typically, we do not see a similar increase in wrist fractures in men over the age of fifty.

Although a wrist fracture can be one of the first indicators that osteoporosis is present, hip fractures are one of the most potentially debilitating fractures; in some cases, they are life threatening due to complications that can occur before or during treatment. *Ninety percent of all hip fractures occur due to a fall,* most often a fall to the side. The hip can fracture in many places, as seen in Figure 1.7 on the next page. (See Figure 3.1 on page 66 for an illustration of how the hip bone [femur] connects to the larger anatomy.)

Why Do We Lose Height as We Age?

Once we get past childhood—when, for many of us, our height was charted by tick marks on the kitchen wall—we assume that our height is set and stable throughout adulthood. Our spine, however, has spacers, or rather discs, that sit between each vertebra and are composed of a thick, fibrous material. These intervertebral discs make up a quarter

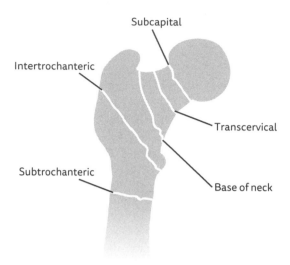

FIGURE 1.7. Fractures in various regions of the femur bone of the hip. Fractures of the transcervical and subcapital regions are the most common.

of the height of the vertebral column. They function as stabilizers and range from ¼ inch to ¾ inch in thickness. The largest are located in the lower spine. When we stand, the discs compress, which results in an average height loss of one centimeter throughout the day. For this reason, we tend to be taller in the morning than in the afternoon or evening. (According to urban lore, some candidates for police or firefighting jobs insist on being measured early in the day so they will meet height requirements.) If you are tracking your own height, it's wise to do so around the same time each day—this will give you the most accurate reading. (*Note:* Because they are done so quickly with equipment that may not be precise, height measurements at doctors' offices can be inaccurate; therefore, it's best to do your own.)

Compression fractures caused by a car accident, or even by landing hard on your buttocks at some point in your life, can result in height loss. Osteoporosis-related fractures of the spine can set the stage for future compression fractures, which could result in total height loss of two to six inches or more over the course of late adulthood.

In addition to compression fractures, other factors that contribute to height loss include:

o *loss of disc thickness in the spinal column that occurs with aging:* This is actually the number-one reason for height loss. When we grow older, the disc material hardens and shrinks. In a healthy young adult the discs in the lumbar (lower back) region can be as thick as ½ inch or more.

o *Deterioration of the joint space between the vertebrae (which includes the intervertebral disc):* This deterioration is called "osteoarthrosis" (also known as "DJD"—degenerative joint disease). DJD can result from a number of inflammatory diseases, including rheumatoid arthritis. It is especially seen in areas of the body and spine that have incurred soft-tissue damage earlier in life and most frequently affects the lumbar spine. Over time, the disc between two vertebrae may become completely flattened, resulting in painful bone-on-bone movements. (Keep reading for more about DJD.)

Osteoporosis and Osteoarthritis: What's the Difference?

The terms "osteoporosis" and "osteoarthritis" are commonly confused. As we stated earlier, "osteoporosis" literally means "porous bone." Breaking the word "osteoarthritis" into its roots yields:

osteo = bone

arth = joint

itis = inflammation

As you can see, then, "osteoarthritis" means "inflammation of the joints." Figure 1.8 on the next page shows a close-up of a spine that is affected by osteoarthritis.

The term "degenerative joint disease," mentioned above, provides a good description of the condition of the joints. It can involve any joint in the body, from the hips to the knees to the vertebral spinal column. When a joint with DJD (also known as osteoarthrosis) develops inflammation, it becomes osteoarth*ritis*.

Osteoporosis, as you learned earlier, affects the bones themselves, not the joints. It is possible to have osteoarthritis without having osteoporosis, but you can also have both of the conditions simultaneously.

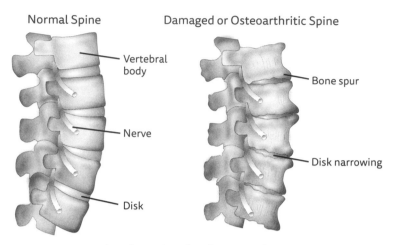

Normal Spine   Damaged or Osteoarthritic Spine

Vertebral body

Bone spur

Nerve

Disk narrowing

Disk

FIGURE 1.8. Lumbar spine showing normal joint spaces on the left and osteoarthritis of the spine on the right

Are Adults the Only People Who Need to Think about Bone Health?

For active children who seem to thrive on risky activities like scaling to the tops of trees, breaking a bone is almost a rite of passage or badge of honor. Generally, however, resilient young people are expected to endure spills and falls without breaking their bones.

Studies on fractures in the young reveal disturbing trends:

o Fracture rates rose 42 percent among those under age twenty between 1969 and 2001. Rates for boys went up 32 percent, and for girls 56 percent.

o Among children ages nine to twelve, fewer than one in ten girls and only one in four boys are at or above their adequate intake of calcium, according to the National Institutes of Health.

Diets filled with soft drinks, sugar, and processed carbohydrates instead of foods rich in calcium and magnesium—plus a lack of the sunshine vitamin, vitamin D—are cited by researchers as some of the reasons for these dismal statistics. In addition, few children in the United States get enough exercise. What's key about these findings is a fact you learned earlier in this chapter: We develop most of our bone before age eighteen. If young people fail to get enough bone nutrients, they will almost certainly have lower than normal peak bone mass, as well as other health problems later in adulthood. These statistics underscore the vital importance of paying attention to bone health in our children.

How Many People Are Affected by Osteoporosis?

Osteoporosis currently affects millions of people in the United States, and it will most likely impact millions more in the future. The U.S. Preventive Services Task Force goes so far as to estimate that as many as one in two women and one in five men are at risk for an osteoporosis-related fracture during their lifetime.

The National Osteoporosis Foundation reports that in 2012 ten million people in the United States had osteoporosis—eight million women and two million men.

Finally, one other statistic from the foundation is especially important to consider: Almost thirty-four million people in the United States have low bone density, which puts them at risk for osteoporosis and fractures in future years. This means that more than 50 percent of people age fifty or older could develop osteoporosis. With the growing population of aging baby boomers, this percentage will almost certainly increase, as the number of people in the United States who are over age sixty is expected to hit 92.2 million in 2030 and 112 million in 2050.

Despite the huge numbers of people whose lives are impacted by osteoporosis, however, the condition continues to be overlooked by patients and doctors alike. Surgeons who repair fractures in older adults may fail to talk to them about the possibility that osteoporosis might be an underlying cause. At the same time, some patients do not consider themselves to be at risk for the condition because they retain the common misconception that it occurs only in the very old. Several studies conducted in 2002 and 2003 showed that the majority of patients with hip fractures were neither diagnosed nor treated for osteoporosis. Further, the Centers for Disease Control reports that although one out of three adults age sixty-five or older falls each year, fewer than half talk to their health-care providers about the fall. And the National Bone Health Alliance estimates that only 20 percent of people over age sixty-five who break a bone get a test or treatment for osteoporosis.

Osteoporosis has been called a silent disease because it can develop for years without your being aware of it. Remaining silent about this condition yourself, however, is not the best approach to caring for your health. It is important for you to speak up, ask questions, and learn as much as you can about your own susceptibility to osteoporosis and fractures.

Are Hip Fractures Declining in Number?

One silver lining behind the cloud of osteoporosis statistics hovering over a large portion of the U.S. population can be found in several studies showing that the number of hip fractures is declining. Consider these reports:

o In 2009 the *New York Times* cited two studies documenting a decrease in hip fracture rates:

   1. Dr. Stephen H. Gehlbach of the University of Massachusetts-Amherst reported a 20 percent decline in the age-adjusted hip fracture rate for men and women between 1993 and 2003.

   2. A Canadian study published in the *Journal of the American Medical Association* found that hip fracture rates fell by 32 percent in women and 25 percent in men from 1985 through 2005.

o In 2012 the American Society for Bone and Mineral Research released findings from a study of Medicare beneficiaries conducted by researchers at the University of Alabama at Birmingham, who stated, "[H]ip fracture incidence has declined among Caucasians in the United States since 1995." Further, a "significant decreasing trend in hip fracture incidence from 2000/2001 to 2008/2009" was also present in white women and men.

So far, researchers cannot point to specific reasons for the apparent decline in hip fractures. Some attribute the trend to a decrease in the numbers of elderly women who lived through the Depression. Earlier (pre-1997) statistics included women who had experienced food shortages in the 1930s and as a result most likely failed to develop adequate bone mass in their youth, which in turn led to increased fractures.

While some researchers acknowledge the positive aspects of the downward trend in hip fracture rates, others express concern that it could lead to a false sense of security about fracture risk. Even if hip fracture rates do not rise in the foreseeable future, an increase in the population of older adults means that the problem will affect vast numbers of people. The American Academy of Orthopaedic Surgeons estimates that by 2050 the annual number of hip fractures will hit 650,000—which translates to almost 1,800 hip fractures a day.

As researchers continue to sort out the data on hip fracture rates, perhaps the best thing you can do is reduce your risk of falling. As the Centers for Disease Control and Prevention (CDC) warns:

"More than 90% of hip fractures are caused by falling— most often by falling sideways onto the hip."

Does One Fracture Lead to Another?

The International Osteoporosis Foundation reports that "…approximately half of all people who have had one osteoporotic fracture will have another, with the risk of new fractures increasing after each fracture." The foundation also points out that the risk of future osteoporotic (non-trauma-related) fractures is particularly high for those who do not get diagnosed or treated for osteoporosis. To promote bone health, the foundation sponsors World Osteoporosis Day to draw attention to its "Stop At One" program, which recommends clinical assessments and treatment for those over age fifty who have had a fracture. Similarly, the 2Million2Many campaign expresses the importance of bone density testing for middle-aged adults with the slogan "If it's 50+ fracture, request a test." (For more information on these efforts, check the following websites: www.iofbonehealth.org and www.2million2many.org.)

One thing to keep in mind about the statistics on repeated fractures, however, is that some studies do not identify whether the initial fracture was caused by a trauma such as an automobile accident. People who break a bone in a car crash during their twenties are not necessarily at increased risk for fractures as older adults. Still, if you have experienced a fracture at mid-life, it is very important to have a bone health assessment that includes a bone density test.

Preventing Falls and Fractures

As you will learn in forthcoming chapters, there is a lot we can do to prevent fractures and improve bone health. One of the most important ways to accomplish these goals is to avoid falling or some other mishap that can result in a broken shoulder, hip, toe, wrist, or vertebra. How important is this kind of prevention? As noted above, the overwhelming majority of hip fractures—90 percent or more—result from falling!

Many practical measures can be implemented to help prevent falls, and a number of them are highlighted in the section on tips for avoiding falls in Chapter 11. That chapter will also offer advice for those who want to stay active in their later years without sustaining fractures. For now, however, I want to give special attention to the most important thing you can do to keep from falling down and possibly fracturing your bones:

Be mindful of your movements.

It may seem obvious or simplistic to point out that it is important to pay attention to where you step in order to avoid missteps. But it is surprising how often people admit that they took a tumble because they were simply not paying attention to what they were doing or where they were walking. In our hyperactive society, it is easy to become preoccupied and distracted. When a lack of attention combines with the slower reflexes and poorer eyesight of older age, it becomes easier to fall. Practicing mindfulness—a state of being relaxed yet focused—can help you stay aware of your surroundings while being centered in your body, so you are less likely to lose your balance or trip over something that is in your path.

I had a patient who told me that she had fallen several times in a single year while walking in her neighborhood. In response to my question about why she fell so often, she replied, "Because the sidewalks in Berkeley are so bad!" It's true that Berkeley sidewalks can be uneven and full of cracks. But when I take a walk on an uneven sidewalk, I make it a special point to watch where I'm going and to lift my feet. To avoid falls and fractures, it's important to keep your mental state as balanced as your body. Being mindful and aware of your movements is not the same as being worried that you could fall at any moment. Granted, it can be difficult to keep that balanced view when you've been diagnosed with osteoporosis or have already sustained a low-impact fracture. When you are mindful, you stay in touch with your body and are able to move appropriately and without fear. Everyone can learn from the example of another of my patients who walks with a brace on one leg. She has a condition that impacts her balance. At one point I asked her about falling, and she replied, "I *never* fall. I walk slowly and pay attention."

○○○○○

The statistics on fractures clearly show that aging and osteoporosis put many people at risk for breaking their bones. The data can provide a broad-brush picture of public health issues; however, that picture needs to be narrowed to bring the state of your own health into focus. As stated at the beginning of the chapter, it's important to remember that you are a unique individual, and many people, including those with osteoporosis, live into their later years without fracturing their bones. Your personal health history must be carefully evaluated to determine the appropriate steps for diagnosing and treating potential bone problems as you age. Keep in mind, too, that you can improve bone health at any age by addressing nutrition, exercise, and digestive issues. And remember, being proactive—what I call being your own health advocate—is the best way to ensure you get the information you need to make informed decisions about your health.

Fracture Fears: My Story

I had to confront my own fears about the possibility of breaking a bone when I was diagnosed with borderline osteoporosis in my mid-forties. But I worked through those fears. First, I realized that in my particular situation my immediate fracture risk was minimal. In fact, I recognized that reaching the age of forty-five with no fractures or other major risk factors meant that my bone health was probably good and my personal risk of fracturing easily was low. Today I continue to be athletic; I hike, bike, play tennis, work out at the gym, and run—but I no longer dive for tennis balls or go after a hard shot on the court. When

(cont'd.)

I bike, I ride more slowly and favor side streets with less traffic. When I turned sixty-three, I decided to stop roller-skating. Although I love skating, at this point in my life I'm finding it more important to avoid the risk of sidelining myself with a fracture that could have been avoided. While I participate in a few activities that some of my medical friends think are too risky for me, I am willing to take that measured risk. Each individual must decide what is right for them. If I ever sustained a fragility fracture, that experience would likely change my activity level. I plan to remain active, and I continue to work to maintain and strengthen my bones through diet, exercise, and nutritional supplementation. In terms of medications, I am not personally opposed to taking them when and if it is necessary. I am a strong advocate of the wise use of conventional medicine.

KEY POINTS FROM CHAPTER 1

- Eighty percent of our lifetime bone mass is laid down by the age of eighteen.

- Some women can lose as much as 20 percent of their bone density during the five to ten years just before and after menopause.

- Osteoporosis fractures are considered low-trauma fractures.

- Wrist fractures are often the first warning sign for women that they may have osteoporosis.

- More than 90 percent of hip fractures are caused by falling.

- Nutrition and exercise are key factors in maintaining healthy bone and preventing fractures.

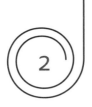

Bone Density Screening: Right Test, Wrong Results?

If your car's fuel gauge is off, the worst that might happen is you'd run out of gas and need a tow—or a battery charge, if the car's electric. But if the tools used to gauge your *health* malfunction, the consequences are much more serious. Unfortunately, when it comes to evaluating fracture risk, bone density testing procedures can be off the mark. And that can result in your getting the wrong diagnosis, the wrong treatment plan, or unnecessary medications.

Consider what happened to Ellen, a woman in her sixties who'd had several bone density tests over the years because of concerns about osteoporosis.

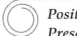 *Positioning Error Leads to*
Prescription for Fosamax: Ellen's Story

Ellen called me from her home on the East Coast after a mutual friend recommended she ask me to assess her latest bone density test. Just listening to her story over the phone, I could tell that something was not right regarding the reported findings of her test. The most recent exam showed that Ellen had lost 7 percent of the bone density in her hip since her previous test a year earlier, but her spine remained unchanged. The discrepancy raised a red flag for me. As a densitometrist, I know that it is highly unusual to see such an extreme loss in the hip, especially within one year.

(cont'd.)

My suspicions were confirmed when I sorted through the stack of paperwork Ellen sent and after I reviewed each of her bone density scans. Comparing the two most recent tests, I could tell that the first technician had failed to position Ellen's hip properly (using a fifteen- to twenty-degree internal rotation), while in the second test the hip was properly positioned.

Why does hip rotation matter during a bone density test? If the hip is incorrectly positioned, errors in density readings of up to 10 percent can occur. That can make the difference in whether or not a doctor recommends medication, as bone loss is a trigger for prescribing drugs. It could also make the difference in whether or not a person is diagnosed with osteoporosis. In Ellen's case, the mistake led to an erroneous report of a 7 percent bone loss, which, understandably, made her very upset.

What's worse, none of it should have happened. In Ellen's first bone density test, the technologist's failure to properly rotate her hip should have been caught and corrected before the report was made—if not by the technologist then by the reporting doctor handling the test. Then, for Ellen's second test, the technologist did rotate her hip correctly, but failed to note the error from the previous test. This is the mistake that resulted in the report of an apparent 7 percent bone loss in Ellen's hip. Compounding the problem, the doctor who wrote the report on the second test results did not catch the mistake either. If the test results were truly showing such a significant change in her bone density, Ellen's own physician should have ordered lab tests to investigate the problem further, but that did not happen; instead, she was prescribed Fosamax, a drug for treating osteoporosis. Believing that the reports were accurate, most medical doctors would likely have done what Ellen's physician did, which was to recommend medications solely on the basis of apparent bone loss.

Once I was able to guide Ellen in getting an accurate bone density reading, we discovered that her bone was stable—meaning no active loss of bone. Additional lab tests verified this finding. To date, she has been able to maintain her bone stability by following a bone-healthy nutrition and exercise program that includes appropriate nutritional supplements—and currently she has no need for osteoporosis medications.

I wish I could tell you that Ellen's case is unusual. But it's not. I see similar bone density testing errors over and over when consulting with my patients. These problems are common knowledge among those trained in densitometry. We all know that preventable mistakes are being made. Why does this happen?

Testing Bone Density: No Expertise Required

Several factors explain why so many bone density tests are fraught with errors. Here are two of the main ones:

1. The technologists who *administer* bone density exams are not always legally required to receive specialized training or certification. Regulations governing bone density testing vary from state to state.

2. Currently there is no legal requirement that the doctors and radiologists who *assess* bone density test results be trained in densitometry, so these professionals may be unaware of how to accurately assess the scan pages for potential pathologies and technical errors. As a result they may rely too heavily on computer-generated reports or on technicians who may not have received adequate training themselves.

Basically, getting certified in the field of bone densitometry is strictly voluntary in many parts of the country. As of this writing it is voluntary for the doctors who write the reports to receive any training, and they are not required to take an exam to demonstrate proficiency. (Keep in mind, densitometry is a subspecialty of radiology, just like mammography.) Few people are aware of the lack of required training, and some physicians whom I've informed of this fact are shocked the first time they hear it.

Many conscientious health professionals do, of course, make the effort to earn certification from the International Society for Clinical Densitometry (ISCD). Other organizations around the country conduct various training programs as well. For instance, members of the American Registry of Radiologic Technologists (ARRT) can fulfill certain training requirements that entitle them to pursue a densitometry certification from the ISCD. And, in California, the Foundation for Osteoporosis Research and Education (FORE) offers coursework leading to a limited license in bone densitometry for technologists.

Completing a certification program, however, is time consuming and costly. Though class instruction time may not be lengthy, the ISCD exams set the bar high for candidates and require them to demonstrate a detailed understanding of the numerous variables that affect bone density test results. In addition, the lack of consistency in the regulations governing professional-level certification weakens the incentives for pursuing training—which means doctors' offices and testing facilities are not always staffed with personnel who can properly conduct and evaluate bone density tests.

What Is Bone Densitometry?

Bone densitometry is a medical imaging technique that is a subspecialty within radiology. As the name implies, it involves the measurement of bone density. Specifically, to evaluate bone mineral density, the technique works by calculating the difference between the amount of radiation absorbed by the patient's hard and soft tissues. This analysis of radiation absorption is why this type of medical imaging is also known as "absorptiometry." A little later in the chapter, you'll read about the main technology used for bone density testing, "dual-energy X-ray absorptiometry" or DXA (formerly abbreviated as DEXA). Because it is a relatively newer field—and because it uses a very low level of radiation—densitometry does not have the same certification requirements throughout the United States as those that govern most types of radiology.

The International Society for Clinical Densitometry (ISCD) offers the following certification programs:

- o *CBDT (certified bone densitometry technologist):* CBDTs perform functions that are somewhat similar to those of an X-ray technician or the personnel who take mammograms. Their work involves positioning patients on the table of a DXA machine, pinpointing the "regions of interest" (areas of the body) being tested, and producing the "diagnostic pages" that are interpreted by a densitometrist. In order to maintain an active license they must be retested periodically or prove that they have earned a certain level of continuing education credits.

- o *CCD (certified clinical densitometrist):* Rather than actually conducting the bone density test procedure—as a densitometry technician would do—CCDs evaluate and interpret the scan results. The densitometrist receives the scanned diagnostic pages from the technologist and first determines if the test was conducted properly; for instance, they check the patient's positioning, the region of interest, etc. After analyzing the scan, the CCD provides a report that includes a diagnosis, and, possibly, recommendations for additional diagnostic tests such as CT scans, X-rays, MRIs, or lab work. The CCD may also make suggestions as to whether or not treatment should be considered. Some densitometrists also review patient scans and offer second opinions or consult with other health professionals on bone density issues. CCDs must be retested periodically or earn required levels of continuing education credits.

Who Gets Trained in Densitometry?

The doctors and radiologists who write the reports after analyzing bone density scans are not required to be specially trained or certified in densitometry, though many have been writing reports for bone density exams since the 1990s, when the testing technology first became widespread. Some doctors, of course, have developed expertise in this area, and because of their experience and/or continuing education are capable of properly analyzing bone density tests—whether they sit for the certification exam or not. Many others, however, do not recognize the complexity of bone density exams and the many details that must be considered to ensure the test results are accurate. For some patients, a doctor's lack of training and/or certification in densitometry can present problems ranging from incorrect diagnosis to the prescribing of unnecessary medications. It's always prudent to ask about a medical professional's level of training or education and, if necessary, to seek additional opinions—perhaps from a certified densitometrist—to make sure you are getting accurate advice about your bone density. To find a list of CCDs in your state, go to the ISCD website: www.iscd.org.

When an imaging facility or a physician's office purchases (or leases) new bone density testing equipment, the manufacturer will provide minimal training to the staff. (Employees hired later may or may not receive any training from the manufacturer.) This type of instruction is not to be confused with the accredited training programs required for a certification in densitometry. In addition, if doctors buy used machines, even the minimal level of training from manufacturers may be unavailable. Then, too, physicians have been known to simply have their untrained front-office staff conduct the tests. This practice is diminishing, but it still exists.

Over the years, I have reviewed cases from various locations around the country, and I have rarely seen reports written by trained densitometrists. On top of that, when I call facilities to ask the technician if they have been trained, most reply, "Yes, the manufacturer trained me"—but again, instructions from the manufacturer are nowhere near the level of education required for a certificate in densitometry. The International Society of Bone Densitometry offers excellent training for technicians and densitometrists that qualifies them to be able to produce a bone density scan and report that have diagnostic value. And the Foundation for Osteoporosis Research in Oakland, California, offers training for technicians only.

As you can imagine, the lack of proper training for people handling bone density assessments can result not only in problems for patients but also in anxiety for the people giving the tests. I will never forget the phone call I received from a young receptionist who wanted to discuss her questions and concerns about testing patients. "I wish the doctor here would send me to get training," she told me, "because I don't know what I'm doing!"

No one should be put in the position of providing or receiving faulty medical tests. That's one of the reasons I felt compelled to write this book. I hope to alert you to the problem and add my voice to those of the individuals working to resolve it. In the meantime, what can you do? How can you and your doctor get the correct information about the condition of your bones?

You'll find answers to these questions throughout the book, particularly in the section in Chapter 3 titled "Steps You Can Take to Get a More Accurate Bone Density Test." First, though, to gain more insight into the issue, let's review a little history of bone density testing. Then we'll look at what happens when the testing goes wrong.

Bone Density Testing with DXA: The Tarnished Gold Standard

When someone sustains injuries following a hard fall off a bike or a crash on a ski slope, it's fairly common for doctors to order X-rays to determine whether any bones are broken. Ordinary X-rays, however, do not provide the information needed to assess bone density and fracture risk. For that purpose, an advanced form of X-ray technology was developed in the 1980s, which today is commonly referred to as DXA. (At one point, the X-ray technology used to measure bone density was abbreviated "DEXA." Whereas "DEXA" may still appear in some publications or websites, this book uses "DXA.")

DXA, which stands for "dual-energy X-ray absorptiometry," sends two low-dose beams of radiation through the body to assess bone mineral density (BMD). In 1994, when the World Health Organization (WHO) decided to use bone density measurements to define osteoporosis, DXA technology began to be viewed as the gold standard for diagnosing the disease. That designation remains widely accepted today. Quite simply, when administered correctly DXA *is* the gold standard.

DXA became the benchmark for measuring osteoporosis because it can provide a reasonably precise measurement of BMD through a painless, noninvasive process that uses minimal radiation. Furthermore, it was seen as a significant advance in the field because prior to its development the diagnosis of osteoporosis was often pronounced only after a fracture occurred.

By 1995 the use of DXA scanners was in full swing; they were found at hospitals, imaging centers, and physicians' offices, including my own office. The new technology also coincided with an upsurge in the marketing of osteoporosis drugs and public awareness of this health problem—particularly among younger women who were increasingly being diagnosed with something called "osteopenia," a condition that today is more accurately recognized as simply "low bone density." The pharmaceutical companies that developed osteoporosis medications in the early 1990s began to place different types of DXA devices in doctors' offices around the United States. Critics charge that this push was designed to promote demand for their products by increasing the number of people getting bone density tests. Often, the devices provided by the drug companies were peripheral machines, which measure only the heel, finger, wrist, or forearm. (Peripheral devices are described in more detail in the next chapter.)

Though DXA screening received the WHO's stamp of approval, the training and professionalization of those giving and analyzing bone density tests did not accelerate at the same rate as the technological advances. This gap in training—as well as inconsistent regulations—has opened the door to countless mistakes in the administration and evaluation of DXA scans, some of which are outlined below (in the section "When DXA Testing Goes Wrong"). See Figure 2.1 on the following page for a graphic representation of one study's estimate regarding the prevalence of problems in DXA testing. As illustrated by the erroneous reports on bone loss described in Ellen's case, the lack of human expertise can turn the DXA "gold standard" into lead.

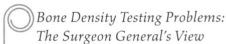

Bone Density Testing Problems: The Surgeon General's View

In a report released in 2004, the office of the U.S. Surgeon General recognized the problems created when health-care practitioners lack sufficient training or certification in densitometry. Titled *Bone Health and Osteoporosis*, the report stated that there is "variability in the ability of technologists to perform the tests, in the training and ongoing certification of technologists, and in interpretation of results by physicians, each of which can undermine the comparability of results." The report went on to say, however, that "despite these limitations, bone mineral density remains the single best predictor of fracture risk available today." Although the state of training is not good, if you have only one bone density test you will be within 5 to 10 percent accuracy in terms of diagnosis.

Trouble arises in determining whether or not you can rely on follow-up tests for diagnostic purposes—that is, to tell you if you are actually losing or gaining bone. You will learn more about this topic in Chapter 3.

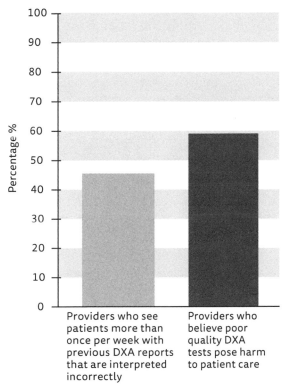

FIGURE 2.1. Bone density reporting errors

Adapted from Michael Lewiecki, MD, FACP, FACE, http://www.projectsin
knowledge.com/osteoporosis/osteoporosis_1/Case-Study-Management
-Poor-Response-to-Bisphosphonate-Therapy.cfm?jn=1894.04

When DXA Testing Goes Wrong

Because DXA testing is considered the gold standard, physicians and patients are often lulled into a false sense of security, thinking that it automatically and consistently provides accurate information for medical decisions. Unfortunately, that is simply not the case. Some problems are inherent in the sensitive DXA machines themselves, while other inaccuracies arise from human errors and testing site practices. This section outlines some of the common reasons for bone density testing mistakes.

Differences in DXA Machines

No two manufacturers produce DXA scans in exactly the same way. In fact, no two machines from the *same* company will produce the exact same results. Because of the inherent differences in all DXA scanners, patients are advised to get follow-up tests on the same machine as the one used for their prior tests. Maintenance of the equipment at testing sites is also essential for precision and accuracy.

Changing the Test Site Changes Results: Connie's Story

Connie received her first DXA scan at a facility near her home. But when she switched to a new health insurance plan, she could no longer get coverage for tests at that facility—which meant she had to go to a new testing center for her second, follow-up test. This created a huge problem, because different DXA machines produce different results, and sure enough, the second test indicated she had lost 6 percent bone density over a two-year period. Connie was so concerned that she decided to spend her own money to return to the first location to be retested. After being rechecked on the original machine, a comparison between tests showed that she had not, in fact, lost bone density.

Rushed Testing

Though bone density testing can be done in relatively short order, the process should not be speeded up unnecessarily. Technicians need time to make sure patients are positioned correctly and that the equipment is capturing the proper images. In some facilities, demands from management can create pressures for technicians to rush through tests, which can lead to inaccuracies. Some of the pressures from management have to do with how little reimbursement they receive for the scans from health insurance companies and Medicare.

Failure to Establish "Least Significant Change" Data

One aspect of DXA scanning that affects results is something known as "least significant change" (LSC). The reality is that there will be variations between two tests on a single patient, even if the same technician conducts the two tests using the same machine on the same day. The LSC is a method of accounting for these variations. Although doing so can be costly, especially for small imaging centers, best practices demand precision assessments in order to include the LSC calculations in the reports. To establish the LSC, fifteen to thirty volunteer patients have two to three scans—one right after the other—on the same machine, by the same technologist. All technicians at the site complete this test, including any newly hired technicians. A series of calculations is used to determine the amount of change between scans from all technicians. The LSC is established for the facility from these data. The test is also a good way to make sure each technician is doing a good job with patient placement and scanning procedures.

The LSC at most DXA sites usually ranges from 3 to 5 percent, which essentially represents the margin of error for a DXA test. That means if a patient is told they have gained or lost 2 percent of their bone density, it is not a reliable number because 2 percent is within the test's margin of error. The LSC will appear on the test report if a facility has established it; however, if the LSC has not been determined, assume it to be about 5 percent. While this news regarding testing reliability may be shocking to some, it is true of most types of testing, including blood and other lab testing. Proper training minimizes testing errors. To learn more about precision assessment, visit the International Society of Clinical Densitometry website (www.iscd .org). They provide help for centers who wish to conduct this test.

Insignificant Changes: Andrea's Story

Andrea's second DXA test indicated that she had lost 2 percent of the bone density in her spine over a five-year period. She had low bone density (−2.3 T-score; see Chapter 3 for a discussion of T-scores) and no other risk factors for fracture. Based on the reported 2 percent loss, her doctor recommended that she start taking a bisphosphonate medication such as Boniva or

(cont'd.)

Fosamax. What her doctor did not mention is that a change of only 2 percent is not statistically reliable in terms of diagnosing bone loss because it is less than the LSC for DXA tests.

Incorrect Positioning of Patients During Testing

Failure to properly rotate the hips (as explained in Ellen's case at the beginning of the chapter) can cause an inaccurate reading. Likewise, to test the lower back, the spine must be centered on the scanning table. In addition, the technician needs to be sure there is a clear view of the vertebrae in the lumbar spine so that all of them are visible on the scan. A skillful technician who double-checks the scanned bone image on his or her monitor during the procedure can eliminate most of these problems. If patients are not in the correct position initially, technicians can reposition them and complete the exam.

In a study published in the June 2008 issue of the journal *Clinical Rheumatology,* researchers' evaluation of 113 DXA reports identified 61 hip images and 94 spine images showing evidence of improper positioning. The report further stated that the spine was not straight in 48.7 percent of the images. The researchers observed, "We found the ratio of invalid positions surprisingly very high. Although this may stem from local technical problems and may not reflect the overall quality of scans in other centers, such misinterpretations would definitely affect clinicians' decisions in an inappropriate way."

Errors in the Selection of the "Region of Interest" from One Test to the Next

As explained in Chapter 1, bone density testing focuses on the lumbar spine (lower back), hips, and forearm. For a follow-up scan the technician must select the exact same area that was tested before to accurately determine whether there has been a significant change in bone density. On newer DXA scanners there is a "comparison feature" to make sure that all of the main components of interest are in the same position as they were in the previous test. However, the comparison feature is not 100 percent accurate, and the technician must still make sure that the proper region is in fact selected. The region of interest should always be the same across tests; however, errors in selection are fairly common with or without the comparison feature.

Technicians Changing the Bone Borders

Sometimes technicians will "redraw" the borders around the edges of the computerized bone image in an attempt to distinguish the skeletal outline from the background. Unfortunately, this practice can "shave off" some of the bone image, which results in calculations that make it seem that bone has been lost when it hasn't. Alternatively, if bone was "cut" from the image in the first test and not in the second one, it will appear as if the patient has gained bone.

In Figure 2.2, in the image on the right, note the arrow pointing to the two lines that form the outline of the bone. You can see how some of the bone area has been shaved off. This mistake will result in an incorrect comparison of the total hip measurement. This type of error should be noticed and corrected by the technologist and certainly should be caught by the reporting doctor.

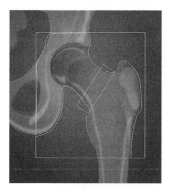 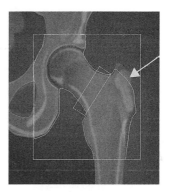

FIGURE 2.2. Incorrect bone area selection (the one on the
left is correct; the one on the right is incorrect)

Inaccurate Comparison of the "Total Hip" to the Neck of the Femur

There are two diagnostic sites in the hip region: the neck of the femur and the area referred to as the "total hip" (see Figure 2.3 on the next page). The femur is the thighbone, and the neck of the femur (sometimes called the femoral neck) is a specific area just below the socket of the hip joint. The femur is thinnest at the neck, which is the most common fracture site in the hip region. When the neck of the femur is compared to the total hip, the discrepancies between the two create an inaccurate result. It is a mistake to juxtapose the measurements of the femoral neck with measurements for the total hip, and this type of reporting error simply should not happen.

It is also important to make sure that the density measurements for the right hip are compared to those of the right hip in a follow-up scan, and that the left hip is compared to the left. Occasionally technicians will erroneously compare the right hip to the left, and vice versa. Current-model DXA machines using updated software generally take care of these types of improper comparisons—but the problem still occurs.

Total Hip and Neck Measurement Areas

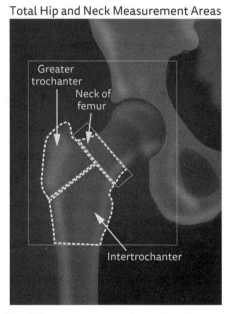

FIGURE 2.3. Total hip measurement includes all three areas in the illustration, which when combined are one measurement. The neck of the femur is also a separate and distinct measurement.

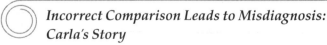

Incorrect Comparison Leads to Misdiagnosis: Carla's Story

Carla came to me seeking a review of her case because a second DXA scan suggested that she had lost 10 percent of bone density within a five-year period. Those results were flawed, however, because they were based on an inaccurate comparison. The reporting doctor had compared the results for the neck of Carla's femur to the results for the total hip from the previous test. As it turned out, Carla had not lost bone at all; in fact, her bone was stable.

Inaccurate Selection of Vertebrae

There are five lumbar vertebrae in the lower back; bone density of the spine is measured by taking an average density of the top four (to view the full spine see Figure 1.5 on page 21). The vertebrae used to measure bone density of the spine are numbered L-1, L-2, L-3, and L-4. Just above them are the twelve vertebrae of the thoracic region, which are numbered T-1 to T-12. Instead of using L-1 through L-4 for calculations, testing personnel sometimes erroneously select T-12 to L-3—that is, they select the bottom thoracic vertebra along with the top three vertebrae of the lumbar spine. This selection will yield an inaccurate result because T-12 cannot be used to determine BMD in the lower back. In a comparison (follow-up) test this mistake can result in an erroneous reporting of bone density loss or gain. Figure 2.4 shows a different type of selection error. In this illustration, the

Comparison Study of the Lumbar Spine

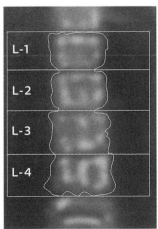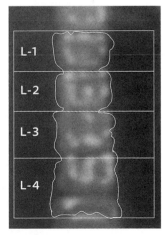

FIGURE 2.4. Correct and incorrect selection of lumbar vertebrae (the scan on the left is correct; the one on the right is incorrect because the bottom of L-4 is not marked correctly, which increases the area of bone and changes the bone density)

image on the left correctly selects L-1 through L-4. By contrast, the image on the right is incorrect because it includes a portion of L-5 in the vertebra labeled L-4. This error yields incorrect results of either bone gain or bone loss. Again, focusing on the correct vertebrae for testing is a fundamental part of densitometry, and failing to do so is the type of mistake that should be easily caught by the technician or certainly by the reporting doctor.

An Average Problem: Jasmine's Story

Jasmine had fractured her L-1 vertebra in a car accident, so her first bone density test did not include that vertebra in the equation for the BMD of her spine. Instead of averaging four of the vertebrae in the lumbar spine, only three vertebrae— L-2, L-3, and L-4—were included. This was the correct way to handle the situation, but when Jasmine was retested, the reporting doctor did not notice that her initial test result was based on the measurements of only three vertebrae. Thus, in the second test, all four vertebrae were included, which threw off the BMD averages used to compare the two tests. Jasmine was told that she had gained bone density, because a vertebral fracture, such as the one that had affected her L-1, typically increases the density of the vertebra. In fact, though, Jasmine had lost BMD. In Jasmine's case, the second DXA test should have been recalculated using the exact same selection of vertebrae that was used in the first test, which would have given her a more accurate comparison.

When Lack of Training Yields Bad Results: An Old Story

Years ago it was discovered that European doctors had a better track record than doctors in the United States when it came to interpreting mammograms. After a full investigation, researchers determined that the likely reason for the discrepancy was because doctors in Europe were required to be fully trained and tested in mammography, while U.S. doctors were allowed to perform the procedure with little or no training. Today, U.S. doctors are fully trained in this specialty, which helps reduce reporting errors.

 How Could I Have Lost 10 Percent of My Bone in One Week? My Story
In the early 1990s, when DXA was still quite new, a colleague who had acquired a scanner asked me if I wanted to use it to check my BMD. Although I had no reason to suspect that I had bone-health problems, after having the test I was told I had the condition called "osteopenia"—meaning I had low bone density in my hip and lumbar spine. I kept up a brave face when he gave me the news, but I remember a tearful drive home as I sadly contemplated a future in which I might not be able to jog, roller-skate, or participate in many of the other physical activities I enjoyed. One week later, after I'd had a little time to digest the initial diagnosis, I decided to be retested at a different facility. This test site used a different brand of machine, and the second test showed that the bone density of my hip was 10 percent lower than it was determined to be during my first test—a result that put my new diagnosis in the borderline-osteoporosis range!

What in the world was going on? How could there be such a huge difference from one test to the next in the space of a week? Even though everyone I knew was touting the DXA test as the gold standard for bone density measurements, I was infuriated by the procedure, which seemed to be so inconsistent. That's when I decided to get to the bottom of the issues surrounding osteoporosis and DXA testing technology—not only for myself but also for my patients. What I learned taught me to be skeptical of BMD results.

As it turned out, the big discrepancy in my readings had to do with inconsistencies in the databases used by the two different manufacturers. In the late 1990s the problem was uncovered, and the particular testing error I experienced has since been resolved—but the fact remains that you cannot accurately

(cont'd.)

compare bone density scans from two different manufacturers. Today more doctors are aware of this fact; however, I still see cases where the doctor sends patients to a different facility for follow-up tests. Because the scanners at the various testing facilities can be made by different manufacturers, patients should obtain all of their BMD tests at the same facility, if possible.

DXA Testing Limitations: False Positives and False Negatives

Many types of medical testing can produce both false positive and false negative results, and DXA scans for BMD are no different. A false positive result indicates a condition or health status that does *not* exist; a false negative result fails to recognize that a condition or change in health status *does* exist. In this chapter we have covered many situations in which technical errors or reporting errors can result in false positive or false negative results. Here are a few more examples to be aware of.

False Positives

One factor that can produce a false positive BMD reading is a person's stature. In terms of bone density, those with a small build are not the same as the average twenty-six- to twenty-nine-year-olds who comprise the population group used as the benchmark for evaluating fracture risks. That means people with smaller builds and who have smaller bones are more likely to be diagnosed as having low bone density or perhaps borderline osteoporosis, while in fact their BMD might actually be normal for them (even if it is "low" when compared to that of an average benchmark group). This does not mean we should ignore low bone density in small-boned people. When small-boned people measure positive for low bone density or osteoporosis, at least part of the low bone density could be because they have smaller bones. You will learn more about this in Chapter 3.

Because standard DXA measurements of BMD may produce false positive results for those with a small stature, some doctors recommend these patients get tested via QCT, which stands for "quantitative computed tomography" and is similar to a CT (or CAT) scan. I do not generally make this recommendation because of the higher degree of radiation exposure from a QCT test. (You'll find more on this topic in the section on bone-testing options in the next chapter.)

False Negatives

Suppose the DXA report shows that the lumbar spine (lower back) appears to have normal bone density, but also reveals evidence of osteoporosis in the hips. In this case, it is possible that the bone density of the lumbar spine is also in the osteoporosis range. It is more common, particularly for women in their fifties, to lose bone density in the spine before they do in the hips. One reason why an individual may show good BMD in the spine but osteoporosis in the hips is because she or he may have osteoarthritis in the lumbar spine. Osteoarthritis can cause a false elevation of bone density, producing a BMD reading that is higher in the spine than is actually the case.

It is well known that different body sites produce different BMD readings, a phenomenon referred to as "site discordance." Inconsistent readings between body sites can indicate false negative or false positive results, so they should be scrutinized carefully. Trained densitometrists can typically sort out these variances and alert the treating doctor about his or her thoughts regarding the possible causes for differences, especially if there is a potential problem that needs further investigation.

Learning about the problems associated with bone density testing can be discouraging for some people and produce anxiety in others. Let me reassure you that it *is* possible to get accurate bone mineral density measurements (and accurate professional advice) to help guide your health decisions. In order to do so, however, you need to know about the negative aspects of BMD testing, and that is why this chapter has focused on those issues. In the next chapter we'll look on the positive side, and you'll find out what happens when DXA testing is conducted properly.

KEY POINTS FROM CHAPTER 2

o When done correctly, bone density tests provide an important piece of information regarding your bone health.

o Errors in bone density testing are common.

o For a more accurate follow-up comparison, bone testing needs to be done on the same (exact) machine.

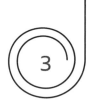

Obtaining the Best Bone Density Test

On one hand, research studies have found that the DXA bone density test is a technology that offers a good level of precision and a proven ability to predict fracture risk. On the other, as seen in Chapter 2, DXA test results can contain significant errors that lead to improper diagnoses and inappropriate recommendations for medications.

If you've read the previous chapter's warnings about the potential problems associated with DXA technology, you might be thinking that I don't recommend this testing procedure. That is not the case. In fact, medical tests of all kinds are often inaccurate, and the problem of potential errors is not specific to bone density testing. My position is this: DXA testing is highly useful *when it's in the right hands*. And those "right hands" include not only technicians and health practitioners who conduct proper tests and produce accurate reports, but also—and most importantly—doctors who balance DXA results with their overall assessment of a patient's bone health before reaching conclusions about treatment.

On the positive side, your first DXA scan provides, at minimum, a baseline bone density measurement—information that gives you a significant piece of the whole, complex picture of your bone health. Even if a test is slightly off, it can still alert patients with low bone density (osteopenia) or osteoporosis that they may need further testing and evaluation.

In addition, while it's easy to have good intentions about eating healthy foods and engaging in exercise, it's just as easy to avoid putting those good habits into everyday practice. Getting the test and receiving a low bone density reading or a diagnosis of osteoporosis can be a motivating factor for people to do whatever they can to build and maintain stronger bones.

There is, of course, the possibility that some who could benefit from the test will decide not to schedule one once they learn about the problems associated with it. That is not my intent. I do not want to discourage anyone from being tested (especially individuals with risk factors for osteoporosis, as discussed in the next chapter). Instead, I want to ensure that those who are tested receive accurate results, so that they and their doctors can make informed health decisions. Along these lines, I fully support the efforts of the International Society for Clinical Densitometry (ISCD) to ensure that bone density technologists and the doctors who analyze and write DXA reports are properly trained and certified.

The bottom line: DXA testing is the gold standard, it yields very important information, and according to the National Institutes of Health, DXA results are the single most important predictor of whether a person will have a fracture in the future. It is a valuable tool, as you have learned, but by no means a perfect one.

Because bone density testing is not perfect, you'll need to take steps to ensure that you get the best results possible. Those steps are explained later in this chapter. To begin, it's helpful for you to understand what you can expect to learn from a bone density test, so that's what we'll look at next.

DXA Testing: A Recap

This section contains a brief recap of bone density testing basics. "DXA" is the abbreviation for "dual-energy X-ray absorptiometry." The DXA test is used to measure BMD, or bone mineral density.

DXA systems:

- o vary from one manufacturer to the next (which explains some of the discrepancies in test results)

- o expose the patient to a very low level of radiation (significantly less than they would get from a mammogram or chest X-ray) o need to be maintained by the facility that uses them—system software needs to be updated and system hardware needs to be serviced regularly to ensure the most accurate test results

Bone mineral density: B M D

o is the strongest predictor of future fracture risk

o accounts for one very significant aspect of overall bone strength

o refers to the concentration of minerals (such as calcium) and other materials within a bone or section of bone

o should be maintained at a certain level to ensure the structural integrity of the skeleton

Bone mineral density is calculated by dividing the bone's mineral content by the area of bone measured. DXA machines calculate bone mineral density by measuring the difference between the amount of radiation absorbed by the patient's hard and soft tissues and the amount of radiation that passes through the body. The machine then uses these measurements to perform mathematical algorithms that calculate BMD results. The denser a patient's bones, the more radiation is absorbed; conversely, the less dense a patient's bones, the more radiation passes through.

Test Results: What's the Score?

Once the DXA scanner measures the bone's absorption of X-ray radiation, it assigns a numerical score to the results. These numerical results are expressed as T-scores and Z-scores. The only scores that are used to diagnose osteoporosis are the ones acquired for four specific vertebrae from the lumbar spine (L-1–L-4), total hip, neck of the femur, and mid-shaft of the forearm (referred to as the "33 percent radius" or the "⅓ radius").

To figure out your T- or Z-scores, your BMD is compared to the BMD of other people in a database. Following are definitions that explain the fundamental difference between a T-score and a Z-score:

o *T-score*: a number representing a comparison between your bone density and the average bone density of *people of the same gender age twenty-six to twenty-nine* o *Z-score*: a number representing a comparison between your bone density and the average bone density of *people of the same gender and age*

For example, if you are a sixty-year-old woman, your T-score compares your BMD to the average BMD of a control group of women in their late twenties. Your Z-score gauges your BMD against that of other sixty-year-old women.

T-scores are unique to DXA testing, and they tend to be confusing and misunderstood. The T-score was invented for osteoporosis and is not used in other diagnostic models.

As with other types of statistical tests, bone density results are measured in terms of "standard deviations," which is abbreviated as "SD." For our purposes, SD describes how much your results vary from the average results for the entire population group you're being compared to. Depending on the information source, each standard deviation from the BMD average is said to equal a 10–12 percent difference in bone density. For the purposes of this book, each SD represents a 12 percent increase or decrease in BMD.

To illustrate: A T-score of –1 means your results are one SD *below* average—and this means, in turn, that your measured BMD is 12 percent below average. Likewise, a score of –2 means your results are two SD below average and your BMD is 24 percent below average. As you can see in Table 3.1, a T-score of –1 or higher is within the normal range for BMD.

T-Score Basics

As described above, the T-score compares an individual's bone density to the average bone density of adults of the same gender age twenty-six to twenty-nine. This comparison provides a valuable perspective for the individual being tested, as the BMD of people in their twenties is at its highest, generally speaking. The T-score gets the most attention from doctors and patients because it is the primary criterion used to diagnose low bone mass or osteoporosis, and in some cases it serves as a justification for prescribing medications.

When is the T-score used to diagnose osteoporosis? A diagnosis of osteoporosis is made when the T-score for the lumbar spine (L-1 to

L-4), neck of the femur, total hip, *or* forearm is –2.5 or lower in the following populations:

o women or men age fifty and over

o postmenopausal women, regardless of age

Table 3.1. T-Score Table

Bone Mineral Density Level	T-score	% of BMD
Normal BMD is no more than one standard deviation (SD) lower than the BMD of the average young adult.	–1 or better	12% below average or better
Low BMD (sometimes called osteopenia) BMD is between 1 and 2.5 SD below that of the average young adult.	–1.1 to –2.4	13.2% to 28.8% below average
Osteoporosis BMD is 2.5 or more SD below that of the average young adult.	–2.5 and lower	30% or more below average
Severe ("Established") Osteoporosis: BMD is more than 2.5 SD below that of the average young adult *and* there have been one or more fragility fractures.		

How are ethnic and racial differences accounted for? When developing T-scores in the early 1990s, the World Health Organization (WHO) based its BMD measurements on those of young, healthy white women, in part because osteoporosis primarily affects white females, and there were insufficient data for the WHO to develop assessments of other ethnic groups at that time. Regardless of ethnicity, T-score calculations compare a woman's BMD to the bone mass of white females age twenty-six to twenty-nine. Similarly, all males are compared to young white men. In general, African Americans have about 10 percent greater bone density than whites, and Latinos have about 7 percent more. Those of Asian ancestry are in roughly the same category as whites in terms of bone density. However, for T-score analysis, all ethnicities are compared to either a male or female white database.

What if the T-score is significantly lower than –2.5? Although a T-score of –2.5 or lower is diagnostic of osteoporosis, there is a big difference between the "cutoff" score of –2.5 and scores that are much lower. Generally speaking, the farther a score falls below –2.5, the greater the cause for concern. A T-score of –4.5, for example, indicates a bone mineral density that is approximately 54 percent lower than the BMD of the control group. That is a significantly low reading; a person with a score of –4.5 is at high risk for fractures, based on bone density alone.

A diagnosis of osteoporosis is a definite red flag that should alert doctors to fully assess the patient to rule out secondary causes for the low bone density. The lower the score, the greater the possibility that a serious underlying problem (such as a nutritional deficiency or disease of the kidneys or parathyroid glands) is resulting in bone loss.

As Table 3.1 below illustrates, a T-score of –1 or better is considered normal for BMD; a reading between –1 and –2.5 indicates low bone mass, but not osteoporosis. The diagnosis of osteoporosis is assigned when the T-score is –2.5 or lower. As shown in the table's right-hand column, each whole-unit increase or decrease in the T-score represents a 12 percent increase or decrease in BMD. Your physician may tell you that you have osteopenia. This is not a disease, but a term created by the World Health Organization (WHO) to describe low bone density.

Note: In DXA reports or other documents related to the bone density test, while BMD readings that fall below zero have a negative or minus sign (–) in front of the number, readings above zero do not have a positive or plus sign (+) in front of them. Occasionally, doctors, patients, and others involved in a case forget this fact and may inadvertently assume that a BMD reading without a plus or minus sign in front of it is in the negative category, creating a false diagnosis and other problems. I once worked with a patient who was told she had low bone density because she had a T-score of 2.0. In fact, she was in the plus range. Although this is a rare occurrence, be sure to double-check any reports you receive, and ask your health care professional to verify whether your scores are on the plus or minus side.

Z-Score Basics

The Z-score, as mentioned earlier, compares your BMD to the average for those of your same gender and age group. Here are a few other basics to keep in mind about Z-scores:

- Z-scores are used to assess premenopausal women and men under age fifty.

- A Z-score better than (above) –2.0 is considered normal for one's age.

- When a Z-score falls below –2.0, BMD is lower than normal for one's age. This result should be a flag for further testing to determine if active bone loss is occurring.

The Truth about T-Scores

Two outcomes resulting from the WHO's 1994 review of worldwide data on bone density testing and fracture risk were the establishment of DXA testing as the gold standard for BMD assessments and the definition of osteoporosis in terms of T-scores. In fact, though, T-scores were not intended as a diagnostic tool; instead, they were designed simply as a means to measure the prevalence of osteoporosis in population groups.

As Dr. Michael Lewiecki, former president of the ISCD, describes it, the WHO classification system for BMD measurements "was not intended for use in the diagnosis of osteoporosis in individual patients. However, in the absence of a better yardstick, it quickly came to be used in that fashion." Dr. Lewiecki also points out that the WHO study group working on this issue chose –2.5 as the T-score cutoff for diagnosing osteoporosis because this score "identified approximately 30% of postmenopausal Caucasian women as having osteoporosis, which is roughly the same as the lifetime risk of clinical fragility fractures in this population."

Dr. Susan Ott, professor of medicine at the University of Washington, calls T-scores "confusing" and cites the failure to standardize DXA machines in the early 1990s as the source of the confusion. As she writes in her course materials on bone physiology, "[W]hen the bone density machines became commercial, the different companies would not agree on a standard measurement.... If the companies would have used the same standards, we could always just look at the plain bone density in grams per centimeter, just like we look at cholesterol in milligrams per deciliter.... Unfortunately, that did not happen. Instead, the T-score was invented."

While densitometrists may be able to analyze the raw data for bone density tests, the average patient and his or her treating doctors typically hear about results in the form of T-scores. Certainly, the T-score is helpful, especially when it is significantly low, because that can be an indication of severe osteoporosis. But, as noted elsewhere in the book, it's important to remember that bone mineral density—regardless of where it falls in terms of T-scores (or Z-scores)—is only one aspect of overall bone health. Keeping that perspective, and having your case reviewed by qualified health professionals in the field of osteoporosis and densitometry, is the best way to make sure you are getting an accurate assessment of your bone health.

Osteoporosis Can Be Diagnosed Even When Bone Density Is Normal

Typically, the diagnosis of osteoporosis is made on the basis of T-scores or Z-scores. However, anyone who has sustained an obvious low-trauma fracture can also be defined as having osteoporosis, regardless of the bone density measurement. This is another reason why it is unwise to think of T-score designations as a hard and fast rule, though they can certainly serve as a reasonable and important guideline. Remember, too, that one low-trauma fracture could be a freak accident that may not happen again and may not indicate a severe bone problem. Nevertheless, after a low-trauma fracture occurs, doctors need to monitor the patient carefully. Most commonly, fragility fractures coincide with an osteoporosis diagnosis.

Debunking Osteopenia

You may recall that the T-score table on page 59 includes the label "low bone density" to describe people with T-scores registering between 1 and 2.4 standard deviations below the peak bone mass of the young control population. This label is purposely used alongside the term "osteopenia" because osteopenia is not strictly a medical condition.

In terms of DXA scans, the term "osteopenia" did not really come into vogue until 1992, when it was highlighted during a meeting of the

World Health Organization (WHO). A 2009 National Public Radio story (tellingly titled "How a Bone Disease Grew to Fit the Prescription") featured comments by Dartmouth professor Anna Tosteson, who explained that experts attending the WHO meeting chose the term "osteopenia" to give public health researchers a clear category for their studies—*not* to define a disease state. At the time, Tosteson observed, no one imagined that "people would come to think of osteopenia as a disease in itself to be treated."

Further, Dr. Diane Schneider, a long-time osteoporosis researcher, categorically states, "'Osteopenia' is not a disease," and she advises her patients to take the word out of their vocabularies. The International Society for Clinical Densitometry is working to do just that as it promotes efforts to replace the term "osteopenia" with "low bone density."

Just as "osteopenia" was never meant to define a disease state, so, too, it should not be used to automatically prompt a prescription for osteoporosis drugs. I still get calls from patients who have been diagnosed with "osteopenia" and told they need to start taking medications such as Fosamax or Boniva based on a single bone density reading. You'll learn much more about osteoporosis drugs in Chapter 6, and throughout this book you'll also get a better understanding of what to do if your BMD falls into the borderline area for osteoporosis. The point, for now, is this: A T-score between –1 and –2.4 means you have low bone density, *not* a disease called "osteopenia."

Still, it is important to recognize that a low bone density diagnosis matters, particularly if it suggests active bone loss. For example, let's say you had a DXA scan that resulted in a T-score of –1.2 in the lumbar spine. Two years later the bone density reading for your lumbar spine is –2.3. This later result is still in the low bone density category, but a bone loss of approximately 12 percent has occurred and should be fully evaluated. If you are actively losing bone, you'll want to find out whether it is due to a nutrition problem or some other secondary health condition. If it is, it may be possible for you to stop or slow the loss without resorting to osteoporosis medications.

Furthermore, although the term "osteopenia" came into widespread use in the 1990s when the WHO used it to describe certain DXA test results, radiologists used it prior to that time to indicate any low bone density revealed by ordinary X-rays. But because conventional X-ray machines do not work exactly like the absorptiometry technology in DXA scans, the low bone density that can be seen on an X-ray film must be *significantly* low to be able to see telltale signs of low density that a trained radiologist would diagnose. In order to see the signs on an X-ray, more than 30 to 50 percent low density must be present. For this reason, if the term "osteopenia" appears as part of a diagnosis that is based on a regular X-ray of the spine (or anywhere else in the body), it is cause for concern. Such a finding means the patient most likely has osteoporosis, and further evaluation, including a bone density scan, is necessary.

The fine distinctions between an X-ray and a DXA scan may be confusing to some, so simply remember this: If you see the word "osteopenia" on a report of a *regular X-ray or any other diagnostic imaging, including MRI or CAT scan,* have a serious discussion with your doctor as soon as possible. But if "osteopenia" is described on a report you receive after a *DXA scan,* it means you are in the low bone density category, not that you have osteoporosis. (It also means that the person who wrote the DXA report was not likely trained in densitometry, because densitometrists are encouraged not to use osteopenia as a diagnosis for BMD and instead to report *low bone density.*)

What Happens During a DXA Test?

The DXA test is a simple one for most people. It involves no injections of any kind. It only requires you to lie on a table on your back with straight legs or, sometimes, bent knees. Once you're on the table, the technician positions you for the scan and sets the computer to make the appropriate calculations. You will be asked to remain still and not breathe for a few seconds while the arm of the machine passes over the area being tested.

At some facilities you may not have to change into a patient gown—but, ideally, you should do so because a gown eliminates the possibility of metal items in your clothing interfering with the scan results. For the same reason, leave jewelry at home (or remove it before the test). Avoid taking calcium supplements the day before the test, because undissolved pills can add to the bone density measurement if they are lodged in an area of your intestines that overlaps the bones.

The DXA machine automatically generates diagnostic pages that contain details about the areas tested as well as small images that look like miniature X-rays. Once the technician has completed the scan, the computer-generated results, including the small X-ray images, are given to the reporting doctor, ideally a densitometrist. The doctor should review the diagnostic pages meticulously since the machine is unable to account for some of the more detailed data in the preliminary diagnoses it provides. The reporting doctor generates a report of his or her diagnosis and recommendations, which is sent to the health care professional who ordered the DXA for you (typically your primary care physician) and to any other practitioners for whom you request a copy. It is crucial that the diagnostic pages—that is, the pages that are generated by the DXA computer—be included in the information that you and/or your doctor receive. You can see examples of diagnostic pages in the Appendix at the end of the book.

Increasingly, imaging centers are including a ten-year fracture risk calculation as part of their DXA reports. This calculation is separate and distinct from the bone density reading, and it can be made automatically in centers that use FRAX assessment software as part of the testing process. FRAX—which stands for *fracture risk assessment tool*—was developed by European doctors to complement BMD testing; it is discussed in the next chapter.

See Figure 3.1 on the next page for an illustration of the parts of the body that are typically evaluated during a DXA scan: the hip, the lumbar (lower) spine, and the forearm. The rest of the section provides an overview of what happens during DXA testing of these three areas and summarizes some of the issues surrounding BMD measurements of the individual areas. It may also provide you with a little more insight into your anatomy.

 Bone Scans and Bone Density Scans: What's the Difference?

A bone scan is very different from a bone density scan, but it's not uncommon for people to use the terms interchangeably in

(cont'd.)

everyday conversation. As explained above, a typical bone density scan using DXA technology is a noninvasive process that does not involve injections. A bone scan, by contrast, requires a radioactive substance to be injected into a vein in the arm. Radiation imaging is then used to produce an image of the area of bone where problems are suspected. Although bone scans are used to diagnose certain bone conditions, they are not used to diagnose osteoporosis.

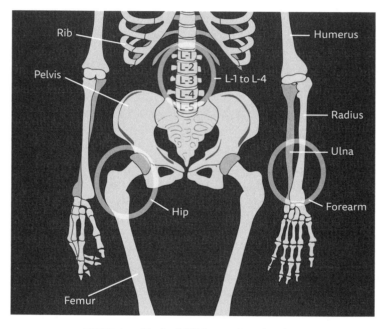

FIGURE 3.1. Typical DXA test sites: lumbar spine (L-1 to L-4), hip, and forearm

Testing the Femur Bone of the Hip

As described in Chapter 2, determining bone density of the hips includes measurement of two diagnostic areas: the *total hip* as well as of the *neck* of the femur. (The femur is the large thighbone that connects to the pelvis.) Some patients get confused by doctors' comments about bone density measurements in the "neck." BMD is only measured at the neck of the femur, in the hip area, not in the neck bones that hold up the head and skull.

It is the technician's job to make sure you are positioned correctly. You may recall from Chapter 2 how important proper positioning is. For the best results, the feet should be positioned in a device that provides a fifteen- to twenty-degree internal rotation of the hip (see Figure 3.2).

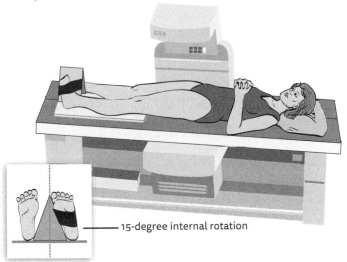

15-degree internal rotation

FIGURE 3.2. Testing the hip

If for some medical or physiological reason you cannot rotate your hips to the degree needed, you can still be tested. When you get a follow-up test, however, your hip should be placed in the exact same position as it was in the previous test, in order to get a more accurate comparison of the two scans.

For follow-up tests: With every new follow-up scan you can remind the technician to look at your prior test and make sure your hip is rotated to the same degree as it was previously.

When the hips are in the correct position (with a fifteen- to twenty-degree internal rotation) on the machine, the *neck of the femur* measures at its lowest bone density level. Too much or too little rotation of the hip will show a false increase in bone density at this site (see Ellen's story, at the beginning of Chapter 2). As discussed in Chapter 2, it is very important that the correct "region of interest" (ROI) be selected for the femoral neck and for the total hip (refer back to Figure 2.3 on page 48). There are many nuances that should be looked at and confirmed for correct selection. For example, newer scanners are designed to automatically select specific areas, such as the femoral neck. If that's the case, the technician must confirm that the correct area has been selected; she or he is able to override the automatic selection if s/he sees that it is incorrect. Since the neck of the femur is included in the score for the total hip, the total hip score is also impacted by inaccurate hip rotation.

For follow-up tests: Subsequent BMD tests must use the exact same ROI as was selected in the initial test; otherwise, it will be impossible to make accurate comparisons to assess whether bone density is stable, increasing, or decreasing. Both the technician and the reporting doctor should double-check the ROI on follow-up tests. If the ROI is off, the facility can reanalyze the scan to make a better assessment without the patient's having to come in for another test. (However, for both follow-up tests and initial tests, you may need to be retested if you were not positioned properly.)

Note: The database used by manufacturers of DXA equipment in the United States for BMD readings on the hip is called the NHANES, which stands for the National Health and Nutrition Examination Survey. Each manufacturing company, however, uses its own database for BMD assessments of the lumbar spine (lower back) and forearm. For more detailed information on the NHANES, go to www.cdc.gov, the website for the Centers for Disease Control and Prevention.

Testing the Lumbar Spine

The lumbar area is, basically, the lower back. The lumbar vertebrae are the spine's largest, and they do most of the back's weight-bearing work. The lumbar vertebrae are labeled L-1, L-2, L-3, L-4, and L-5 (but only L-1 through L-4 are analyzed for BMD measurement).

For checking BMD in the lumbar spine, the patient can be positioned with knees either bent or straight, depending on the DXA machine. As is the case for scans of the hip, for lumbar scans the technician makes sure that the spine is positioned properly. Once the scan is complete, newer machines automatically select L-1 through L-4 as the region of interest (refer back to Figure 2.4 on page 49, image on the left). This specific area is used because it provides the clearest view of vertebrae since the ribs, sternum, and sacrum are not in the way to block them. Because vertebrae selection is often the source of errors, as mentioned previously, the technician should make sure that the four vertebrae have been selected properly. L-4 is identified by two main features: It looks like a bow tie, and it is typically even with the crest of the pelvic bones (if they are visible). Identifying the correct vertebrae may sound easy, but in fact it's tricky. This region of the spine can have many types of anomalies, including six lumbar vertebrae (instead of the usual five) and other normal variants that can impact bone density readings—another reason why technicians must be schooled in anatomy.

The diagnosis of osteoporosis is based on the average of the BMD of L-1 through L-4. Using an average is meant to reduce errors; a single vertebra is less representative of the entire spine. But once the scan is produced, the doctor reading it should evaluate the findings to determine whether or not all four vertebrae are in fact reliable for the bone density test—or if, instead, one or two of them should be taken out of (deleted from) the calculation. Ideally, all four lumbar vertebrae are used in the calculation, and no fewer than two are used for diagnosis, so a diagnosis would never be based on the results for a single vertebra. But there are many reasons why all four vertebrae may not be used, because bones can have many individual differences. For instance, osteoarthritis, and the bone spurs that can develop from it, may cause one vertebra to have a much higher (abnormal) BMD than adjacent vertebrae.

Again, if the lumbar vertebrae show no significant anomalies, then the average reading for L-1 through L-4 is calculated and is used to establish the BMD reading for the lumbar spine. But if any of the lumbar vertebrae show a difference in BMD of 12 percent or more above or below an adjacent vertebra, the "outlier" vertebra needs to be deleted from the equation. For instance, suppose a patient has an old (or new) fracture in L-2. A fracture increases bone density, so the L-2 reading should be deleted—which leaves L-1, L-3, and L-4 to be averaged for the bone density score. Note that when there is such a difference between vertebrae, it is possible that a disease process is the cause. In cases of significant differences between vertebrae, it may be necessary to order additional imaging, such as MRI scans, X-rays, or a CT scan to pinpoint a diagnosis.

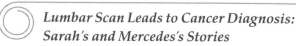

Lumbar Scan Leads to Cancer Diagnosis: Sarah's and Mercedes's Stories

When the DXA scan I provided for Sarah showed that she had a lumbar vertebra whose BMD was 15 percent lower than that of the adjacent vertebrae, I requested a spot X-ray of her spine, which revealed that she had bone cancer. Sarah had had breast cancer many years earlier, and the cancer's metastasis was discovered as a result of the DXA scan performed in my office.

In another case involving a woman named Mercedes, who had very low bone density in one of her vertebra, the DXA scan for that patient was not performed at my office—and the doctor who wrote the report failed to note the irregular vertebra. When I saw the report I ordered X-rays and a CT scan, and the findings resulted in the patient's being diagnosed with multiple myeloma, a form of bone cancer.

Special Issues Affecting Lumbar Spine BMD Readings

When checking the bone density of the lumbar spine, patients with scoliosis (curvature of the spine) or previous surgeries should note the following considerations:

Scoliosis: The spine needs to be as straight as possible to get an accurate bone density reading. If the scoliosis is mild then the technician should make sure that the spine is centered as well as possible on the scanning table. If the scoliosis is significant, the BMD reading of the spine is not reliable, in which case the forearm and hip should be tested. It is always preferable to test at least two diagnostic areas.

Previous surgeries: Past lumbar surgeries also hinder bone density testing. If you have had lumbar surgery, be sure to tell your doctor and the technician—and make certain that any previous surgeries are noted in your file. If you have undergone a surgical procedure affecting your L-4 vertebra, for example, it would still be possible to check the BMD for L-1, L-2, and L-3, but the technician must be aware of the surgery so he or she can notify the reporting doctor.

Scanning Scoliosis: Jane's Story
Jane was a seventy-year-old patient who asked me to review the BMD results she had obtained at a testing facility near her home. Although Jane had severe scoliosis, the facility had provided her with six scans of her lumbar spine over the course of eight years. Scanning the lumbar spine in patients with significant scoliosis is a gross misuse of a DXA test. I can only assume that the technician and the reporting doctor were not trained in densitometry, as it is basic knowledge that accurate results cannot be obtained when the curvature is severe and the spine is not centered on the scanner. Jane's BMD should have been assessed using tests of her forearm and hip.

Testing the Forearm

The forearm, which extends from elbow to wrist, can also be tested to diagnose osteoporosis, but the BMD readings for the lumbar spine and hip are preferable. In certain cases, if the spine or hip cannot be tested for some reason, the forearm may be checked to gather additional data about the condition of a patient's bones. For instance, if someone has had hip replacement surgery, the hip can no longer provide information about bone density, so the forearm would be checked, along with the lumbar spine. Similarly, the forearm measurement is necessary for patients who have had spinal surgery, or who have scoliosis, significant osteoarthritis, or any other condition that might yield inaccurate bone density results.

The forearm has two bones: the radius and the ulna (refer back to Figure 3.1 on page 66). Despite all the names and numbers that appear on the forearm report, for osteoporosis diagnoses DXA testing of the forearm focuses on the diagnostic region referred to as the "⅓ radius" or the "33 percent radius" (see Figure 3.3 on the following page). Generally, the DXA test of the forearm is done on the patient's nondominant arm: the left arm for a right-handed individual, and vice versa.

Remember, in DXA testing the only four areas whose T-scores and Z-scores are used to diagnose bone density are the lumbar spine, total hip, neck of the femur, and the 33 percent (⅓) radius region of the forearm.

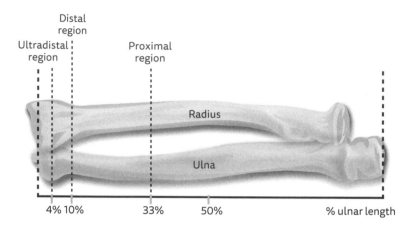

FIGURE 3.3. Testing the forearm
(hand is on the left; elbow is on the right)

A note about site discordance: Each area of the body has a different bone mineral density measurement; thus, there is discordance among the sites used to measure BMD. This is one reason why, for example, a measurement of the heel, a single finger, or the wrist is not to be trusted as representing the bone density of the lumbar spine or hip. To accurately measure BMD it is preferable to test *at least two* areas of the body, not just one. And, ideally, those two areas are the hip and the lumbar spine. As stated earlier, if the measurement for either the spine or the hip cannot be used because of surgeries or other reasons, then the forearm scan is necessary. Some doctors routinely order tests of all three sites to determine BMD and assess fracture risk.

Who Should Get Tested? And When?

One of the paradoxes of bone density testing is that some of the people who most need to be assessed are getting tested the least. Low Medicare reimbursements, for example, are causing some testing centers to close, meaning that a large number of older adults will not be tested (see "Less Medicare Coverage = Fewer DXA Tests?" on the following page). Then, too, other groups of adults may not realize they have certain risk factors for osteoporosis and don't get tested until reaching their mid-sixties, even though catching the condition sooner through early testing could benefit them.

The U.S. Preventive Services Task Force—whose guidelines may have an impact on whether someone's health insurance plan (or Medicare) will pay the cost of a BMD test—recommends osteoporosis screening only for those patients who fit the following criteria:

o women age sixty-five or older

o younger women whose fracture risk is equal to or greater than that of a sixty-five-year-old white woman who has no additional risk factors

Note that the task force makes no recommendations for screening men, although organizations such as the National Osteoporosis Foundation and the International Society for Clinical Densitometry (ISCD) recommend testing for men over age seventy. The more comprehensive recommendations offered by the ISCD suggest testing for the following groups:

o all women age sixty-five and older

o all men age seventy and older

o anyone who has sustained a fragility fracture or a fracture after age fifty

o anyone with a disease, condition, or on medication associated with osteoporosis

o anyone who is considering therapy for osteoporosis, if bone density testing would facilitate the decision

o women who have been on hormone replacement therapy for prolonged periods

o anyone being treated for osteoporosis, to monitor the effects of therapy

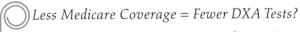

Less Medicare Coverage = Fewer DXA Tests?

In years past, Medicare reimbursement for a DXA test could be as much as two hundred dollars, but Medicare payments for the procedure have dropped considerably, to as low as fifty dollars in some cases. As a result, a number of testing facilities have either closed or are speeding up test times so they can offset their financial

(cont'd.)

losses by processing more patients. Research shows that fewer than 15 percent of Medicare patients receive bone density exams, an indication that those who most need the test are not getting it. Interestingly, hospitals have been known to charge as much as a thousand dollars for the same test, simply because it is done in a hospital setting.

Unfortunately, most of the ISCD screening recommendations listed above are rarely followed, but they are excellent starting points for understanding who should be tested. As the ISCD points out, *anyone*—female or male—who is at risk for developing osteoporosis needs to be tested. (See the comprehensive list and discussion of risk factors for osteoporosis in the next chapter.) In my opinion, it's a good idea for women who have risk factors to be tested prior to menopause. That's because, as you read in Chapter 1, bone loss can be considerable during the years leading to menopause and up to ten years afterward. Women can benefit from testing prior to menopause to establish a baseline measurement for BMD that can be useful for follow-up tests during the menopause transition, when bone loss can occur at a rate of 1–3 percent each year for a five- to ten-year period. Regardless of your sex or menopausal status, early testing and testing for those with osteoporosis-related risk factors can go a long way in helping you to take steps that can *prevent* osteoporosis and needless fractures.

Bottom line:

If you have any reason to think you are at risk for fractures or osteoporosis, do not hesitate to get a bone density test.

It's also important to follow the guidelines presented below in the section "Steps You Can Take to Get a More Accurate Bone Density Test." If you need information about Medicare reimbursements, visit the ISCD (International Society for Clinical Densitometry) website for updates (see Resources).

What sort of timetable should you follow for retesting? I know of patients who have received BMD testing every year, but, generally speaking, follow-up BMD tests are only needed every two years. A certain amount of time needs to pass between tests in order to determine if any loss or gain in bone density falls outside of the margin of error for DXA testing (you may recall the discussion on LSC— least significant change—in Chapter 2). Unless significant bone loss is anticipated over a twelve-month period, annual testing is unnecessary; the two-year guideline is appropriate for most people with osteoporosis, and it also tends to track with most health insurance and Medicare policies. On the other hand, your bone density reading is an individual matter, and every case is unique. It may be necessary to measure your BMD more often depending on your bone-health problems and risk factors.

Steps You Can Take to Get a More Accurate Bone Density Test

In the last chapter and this one, you've learned about what happens when DXA testing doesn't go so well, and you've learned more about how DXA tests function. This information is intended to help you work with your health providers to obtain more accurate DXA tests. The steps outlined below provide additional recommendations that can help you achieve this goal.

o Determine whether there is a facility in your area whose personnel, including the technician and the reporting doctor, are trained and certified in densitometry. If your facility does not have certified personnel on staff, ask about the level of training their technicians have received. If you bring up this issue, the staff may pay closer attention to your assessment. Having credentials, of course, does not guarantee that no mistakes will be made, and some facilities do a good job whether or not the staff has certification. But you stand a better chance of getting an accurate test if you know that staff members have been trained appropriately and have passed exams that demonstrate their understanding of the technology. If you need a bone density test and you don't have access to a facility with certified personnel, get the test anyway. While this suggestion may sound odd given all the caveats I presented in Chapter 2, chances are that your test will be good enough to get a reasonable diagnosis.

o To find a listing of doctors with certification in densitometry, visit the website of the International Society of Clinical Densitometry (ISCD): www.iscd.org.

o If possible, have all of your BMD tests done at the same facility and on the same type of machine—even on the same exact machine if it's available. Each DXA machine manufacturer uses different databases and calibrations, leading to varied results that make it difficult to compare an initial test to a follow-up test if the two are performed on different machines. If, for a follow-up test, you go to the same facility where you went for your first test, ask if they are still using the same machine; they may have purchased a new one. And some facilities have more than one DXA machine; again, if this is the case, make sure you are on the same one that you were assigned to on your first visit. This is important information for your doctor to track, because even with machines produced by the same manufacturer, a 2–3 percent difference in readings is possible.

o When being retested, ask the technician to make sure your hip positioning and rotation match those on your previous test. Skilled technicians who care about their work will already know the importance of positioning patients correctly. But by asking the question, you will alert the technician to pay extra attention to your placement on the scanning table.

o Ask for the "diagnostic scan pages" to be included with the report that will be sent to your doctor (see the examples in the Appendix). The ISCD states that they should always be included with the report, but that does not always happen. The diagnostic scan pages are the ones with the photos that look like small X-rays of the hips and spine. (In some facilities, the front office staff may not understand which pages you are asking about, but the technicians should know, and you can ask to speak to one of them if there is any confusion.) If possible, obtain hard copies (printouts) of the pages. Some facilities provide only a CD containing the images and the report, which you or your doctor can download on a computer. In most cases, however, special software programs are required to print the images, which is another reason to ask the imaging center to print them out for you.

Having access to the scan pages is essential if the densitometrist is to offer a reliable comparison analysis. This will give you important information as to whether or not the tests are diagnostic (reliable) and whether your bone is stable or bone loss or gain has occurred. Always make sure that you get the full DXA report for your records in case you want to get a second opinion. If you've had more than one DXA test, make sure that you have the diagnostic pages from (at least) the two most recent tests.

o The ISCD recommends that you take these practical steps when going in for a bone density test:
  - Are you pregnant? If so, tell the technologist. You should not get a bone density test of the spine if you are pregnant unless it is deemed absolutely necessary. Avoid any radiation until after the baby is born.
  - Eat a normal diet on the day of the test.
  - Take your medications as you normally would.
  - *Do not* take calcium supplements for twenty-four hours before the test.
  - On the day of the test, leave valuables at home.
  - Do not wear jewelry or body piercings to the examination.
  - The test should be performed prior to oral, rectal, or IV contrast studies, or at least seven days after any of these studies.

o Finally, if you are unable to be tested by certified personnel and you are concerned about your results, consider getting a second opinion from a CCD. Again, you can contact ISCD for referrals to densitometry professionals who may be able to review your results.

A note on test anxiety: The actual bone density test procedure is noninvasive and relatively simple, so it should not cause undue stress. Receiving the results from your test, however, may create anxiety, depending on your test results. It is understandable if you become concerned about your health after receiving a diagnosis of low bone density or osteoporosis. But even then, keep in mind the following points: Bone density is only one aspect of skeletal strength; you can do a number of things to improve your bone health; and many people never fracture, even if they have osteoporosis.

Other Bone Testing Devices

DXA technology is the primary method for assessing bone density, but several additional types of bone testing equipment also exist. They include the QCT, the QUS, the pDXA, and others. One way to make sense of this "alphabet soup" is to understand that the equipment for assessing BMD is divided into two main categories: central machine tests and peripheral machine tests. Below you will see how the various tests fall into their respective categories, and I'll also provide information on one test, the vertebral fracture assessment, or VFA, which is in a category of its own. Keep in mind, of course, that new technologies may be developed in future years that could supplant any of these devices.

Central Machine Tests

Central machine tests employ stationary machines that scan bones in the spine, hips, forearm, and, rarely, the whole body. They include DXA and QCT.

DXA—dual-energy X-ray absorptiometry

As noted, DXA machines are the main type used for diagnosing osteoporosis. DXA machines can also do whole-body scans, and they are sometimes used to measure total body composition and fat content (although research is ongoing as to the accuracy of such measurements). DXA testing equipment is primarily available from three manufacturers in the United States: GE/Lunar, Hologic, and Norland.

QCT—quantitative computerized tomography

QCT scans can differentiate between compact and cancellous bone, but this form of computerized tomography requires a much larger radiation dose than DXA. Some doctors order QCT on smaller people since the reading is somewhat more accurate. Because of the higher radiation exposure, I do not typically recommend or order the QCT scan for my patients—unless there is a specific need to use the technology to uncover a suspected medical condition such as cancer. The need might arise if DXA testing shows a significant difference between the densities of two adjacent vertebrae.

QCT is the only other recognized technology that can diagnose osteoporosis with T-scores or Z-scores. Typically, QCT tests only two lumbar vertebrae, L-1 and L-2. The main difference is that QCT can detect the difference between compact (outer layer) bone and cancellous (trabecular) bone (inside microarchitecture).

Trabecular Bone Score (TBS) Testing

In 2013 some imaging centers started including a new measurement when testing with the DXA machine. This measurement, made possible by new software, detects the inside architecture (trabecula) of the bone. Since this technology is relatively new, we don't know yet if it will increase the accuracy of the diagnosis of osteoporosis and fracture risk. For more information on TBS testing, visit my website (www.LaniSimpson.com).

Peripheral Machine Tests

These tests are used to check BMD or bone stiffness in several areas of the body, including the wrist, heel, finger, and shin (tibia), as well as the forearm. Whereas central machines are not portable, peripheral machines are often small, portable units and are sometimes seen at health fairs. Peripheral testing machines include:

pDXA—peripheral DXA (typically forearm)—tests bone density

pQCT—peripheral QCT (typically forearm)—tests bone density

QUS—quantitative ultrasound (of the calcaneus—the heel)—tests bone stiffness

Is there a clinical use for these peripheral devices? Yes, because they can identify people with low bone density who might not otherwise be tested. Besides being portable, the devices are relatively inexpensive. They can detect some cases of osteoporosis, and they may catch the advanced cases. However, they can also miss osteoporosis due to site discordance. Worse, they can give someone a false sense of security, because even if the results from a peripheral machine test are normal or in the low bone density range, a person's BMD in key areas (spine and hip) may be worse.

If you have risk factors for osteoporosis, don't rely on peripheral devices. Make sure to get a DXA scan of the hip and spine. Even when a peripheral test indicates osteoporosis, it's also important to have your hip and spine tested for one very important reason: Peripheral devices cannot be used with any reliability to track the progress of treatment, whether that treatment involves medication or lifestyle changes.

An Example of Site Discordance: My Story

The DXA scan of my wrist shows normal bone density, the one of my hip shows low bone density, and the one of my spine shows osteoporosis. My forearms and wrists are stronger than those of most people because of my years practicing as a chiropractor and doing gardening. My calcaneus (heel) measured by QUS (ultrasound) showed only a minor low bone density, which may be due to my years as a jogger and tennis player. The hip and spine are the most critical areas for determining whether there is a brewing problem or a serious problem because fractures in these regions can be life altering and disfiguring. However, testing the forearm and heel can alert a patient to the need to have her hip and spine tested.

Vertebral Fracture Assessment (VFA)

The VFA, which is separate and distinct from DXA and other tests, is useful for determining the presence of a vertebral fracture. Quite often, people are unaware that they have fractures in their spine because the fractures might not be causing pain or discomfort and they may have occurred at any point in a person's lifetime. Because it is difficult to tell whether fractures are old or new, it is sometimes recommended that certain patients have VFA (see example in the Appendix) in order to establish a baseline reading on the condition of the spine. Then, in the future, if the patient experiences back pain or other symptoms, a follow-up VFA or X-ray can show if a new fracture has occurred. Why is it important to know whether a fracture is new? Because if a low-trauma vertebral fracture occurs, there is a high probability that more will follow.

The VFA can be done on the same DXA machine used to measure bone density; in fact, it can be done at the same time as a BMD test—

but only if the facility has the appropriate computer software for such a test. Many do not.

Who should get a VFA? Though the VFA and the BMD test can be taken together, I do not usually order it for patients unless it is established that they have osteoporosis or other risk factors and a health history that warrants the test. If an adult has a self-reported loss in height of more than 1.5 inches from their tallest measurement, has a stooped posture, or has had previous fractures, it is possible that they may have a vertebral fracture. People who have sustained any fracture over the age of fifty and those who have had a low-trauma fracture are all candidates for a VFA, as are patients with a diagnosis of osteoporosis. While the test does involve radiation, the dose is very low, a fraction of that produced by regular spinal X-rays.

Note: If you have a VFA and receive a fracture diagnosis, you may also need to have an X-ray, especially if you're experiencing back pain. The VFA is good for visualizing the fracture, but an X-ray can help determine if the fracture is old or new (it is always possible that a vertebral fracture was sustained during childhood).

Ask the technician performing your VFA if they have performed one before and, if so, how many times. Patient positioning is very important, especially to view the upper thoracic vertebrae. The arm must be correctly positioned above the head so that it does not overlay the spine. Your asking these simple questions will alert the technician to pay closer attention.

Finally, make sure that you and your treating doctors receive the scan pages for the VFA. And make sure that the reporting doctor graded the fracture if there is one. Most vertebral fractures involve the body of the vertebra, and there is a big difference between a 10 percent compression and a 70 percent collapse. While a low-trauma fracture of any kind is not a good sign, if the vertebra is significantly collapsed, especially if the collapse is new and the vertebra has been subjected to minimal trauma, it is an indication of a more serious bone disease state.

As stated, bone density testing provides only part of the overall picture of your bone health. To fill in the rest of the picture, you need to understand your personal level of fracture risk. That is what we will examine in the next chapter.

KEY POINTS FROM CHAPTER 3

o A diagnosis of osteoporosis does not necessarily mean that you are presently losing bone.

o A diagnosis of low bone density or borderline osteoporosis based on bone density alone, with *no other* risk factors, may not pose much of a risk for fracture.

o Osteopenia (low bone mass) is no longer considered a diagnosis that on its own requires treatment. Instead, it should serve as a wake-up call to take care of your bones.

o Proper positioning during BMD testing is crucial. Poor hip rotation, for example, can show an incorrect gain in or loss of bone density.

o The timeline for follow-up tests for those diagnosed with osteoporosis is about two years.

o For most centers, the least significant change (LSC) is 3 to 5 percent. Therefore, a 2 percent change is within the margin of error and is not reliable.

o Don't wait! Get tested if you have risk factors for osteoporosis.

o Request a complete copy of your test results, doctor's report, and scan pages.

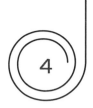

4

Rating Your Personal Fracture Risk

Smoking, high blood pressure, and a family history of cardiovascular disease—these are a few of the well-known signs that may put you at risk for a future heart attack. When it comes to bone fractures, however, the warning signals are not always so obvious or widely recognized. And just as high blood pressure is only one important indication of possible heart problems, so too is a bone mineral density test but a single measure of your potential risk for breaking a bone.

Because BMD reveals only a partial view of bone health, questions that naturally arise include: What *else* poses a risk to the bones? Are there other factors that increase a person's chances of a fracture?

These questions affect literally millions of people. The possibility that massive numbers of older adults could suffer debilitating fractures concerns not only vulnerable individuals and their families, but also public health officials seeking to keep health care costs down while also caring for an aging population around the globe. In grappling with these issues, the World Health Organization (WHO) resolved in the late 1990s to develop a program to identify and assess fracture risks *beyond* the use of DXA testing and T-scores—all with the aim of giving primary care physicians guidelines for treating patients most likely to suffer fractures.

The WHO program resulted in a computerized patient evaluation program known as FRAX, which stands for *fracture risk assessment tool*. This tool—which you can use for free online—helps assess a person's ten-year risk for fractures; the results show the probability of

83

a hip fracture as well as a major osteoporotic fracture (defined for FRAX calculations as a fracture to the lumbar spine, forearm, hip, or shoulder). Initially released in 2008, the FRAX tool has been validated in eleven separate population groups covering one million–plus patient years. It offers models for predicting fracture risk in more than thirty countries.

Despite this pedigree, however, FRAX has its critics and limitations; its shortcomings are addressed in this chapter. For example, FRAX should not supplant a clinician's personal expertise and judgment—and, in my opinion, it should form only one part of a comprehensive assessment of a patient's bone health. In addition to showing you how to use the FRAX tool, this chapter also discusses an alternative: the FORE Fracture Risk Calculator. Finally, the chapter offers a list of risk factors for osteoporosis that are distinct from bone mineral density readings. Becoming aware of these factors will give you a more accurate understanding of your potential for fracturing a bone.

Assessing Risk: Using the FRAX Tool

FRAX is, essentially, an algorithm, which means it is a procedure that walks you step-by-step through a series of questions in order to solve a particular problem. In this case, the goal is to provide an estimate of the probability of your fracturing a bone within a ten-year period.

Available on the Internet as well as through mobile devices, the FRAX tool integrates several well-established clinical risk factors (CRFs) into its calculations for fracture risk. For instance, age is a long-recognized factor that represents an increased risk of breaking a bone. Even if bone mineral density remains the same, fracture risk is higher in the later years than at middle age or younger, so FRAX takes age into account.

To access this tool, search online for "FRAX" or "FRAX + Osteoporosis," or use the following URL for the University of Sheffield in the United Kingdom, which hosts the FRAX website: www.shef.ac.uk /FRAX. The online FRAX assessment is the same one incorporated into some DXA scan reports. If your testing facility does not include it, you can do the assessment yourself by going to the University of Sheffield website.

Selecting the "calculation tool" on the website makes it possible to pinpoint the country of origin for most users; in the case of the United States, this choice can be further refined according to race or ethnic background (white, African American, Latino, or Asian).

Initially, you will fill in the answers for the following basic health information:

- age
- sex
- weight in kilograms (convert pounds to kilograms by dividing by 2.2)
- height in centimeters (convert inches to centimeters by multiplying by 2.54)

Then you will respond using "yes" or "no" to show whether you have the following clinical risk factors for fracture:

- previous fracture
- parent fractured hip
- currently smoking
- glucocorticoid treatment
- rheumatoid arthritis
- secondary osteoporosis
- alcohol consumption, three or more units/day

Finally, if you have had a DXA test to determine your bone mineral density levels, you will be able to select the type of machine that was used. Then you can input your results for *only* the femoral neck. You can enter the score in gm/cm^2 (grams per square centimeter) or the T-score.

Once this information is entered into the program and the "calculate" function is selected, the program shows, in percentage terms, the ten-year probability of both a major osteoporotic fracture and a hip fracture. For example, the risk for a major osteoporotic fracture could read "7.6%," while for the hip it might only be "0.7%." In this example, both readings fall into the "low risk" category.

Note: FRAX can be used even if you do not have a bone density result.

Understanding FRAX Results
and Recommendations

As noted above, the FRAX tool gives users a reading based on an assessment of their ten-year risk for hip fractures as well as major osteoporotic fractures. The probability of experiencing these fractures can vary from one country to the next, and, of course, the tool does not account for all individual differences. Originally, FRAX was intended for doctors and patients to have a guideline regarding whether or not medications should be considered. The guideline is to consider medication if the risk for a hip fracture is 3 percent or more, or the risk for "other" major fractures is 20 percent. This arose out of concern that most doctors prescribing the medications needed a benchmark.

Another way that you might see fracture risk expressed is divided into three categories: low, medium, and high risk. Here is a *ballpark* estimate of the risk for an osteoporotic fracture in each of these categories for a ten-year period (these categories apply to postmenopausal women and to men over age fifty):

- o low risk—less than 10 percent

- o medium risk—between 10 and 20 percent

- o high risk—above 20 percent

Because the FRAX tool was initially designed to help physicians and their patients choose treatment options, FRAX results can have an impact on decisions about osteoporosis medications. The National Osteoporosis Guideline Group (NOGG), in the United Kingdom, and the International Osteoporosis Foundation use the general FRAX risk categories (low, medium, and high) to offer treatment guidelines to clinicians. The U.S. Preventive Services Task Force and the National Osteoporosis Foundation also include FRAX results in their treatment recommendations.

The following treatment guidelines were developed by the NOGG. If you've obtained your FRAX results, whether on your own or through your health-care provider, these recommendations may well apply to you. I've included them here so you will know what doctors are likely to recommend.

o *Low risk*: Clinicians are advised to reassure the patient and re-assess him or her in five years or less. Patients are also provided with lifestyle advice about diet and exercise, but medication is not required.

o *Medium risk*: Clinicians are advised to measure BMD and re-calculate the fracture risk to determine whether an individual's risk lies above or below the intervention threshold. A DXA scan is usually indicated. After the DXA test, fracture risk is reassessed, and the decision is made as to whether medication is needed.

o *High risk*: Clinicians are advised that patients can be considered for treatment without the need for BMD testing, although such testing may sometimes be appropriate, particularly in younger postmenopausal women. A clinician will likely recommend treatment for patients who are at high risk for fractures.

Later in the chapter we will look at FRAX drawbacks. The tool does not take certain risk factors into account—which means it will miss any number of people who need further assessment or treatment, or it may overestimate fracture risk based on the generalized questions that are asked. Like a BMD reading, FRAX results should be regarded as *only one* piece of information that can be incorporated into your bone health picture.

Professionals' Views of FRAX

The commentary below, by Judith Brenner, MD, gives several ex-amples of how different variables affect fracture risk as measured by the FRAX tool, and it also explains how doctors might apply these results to treatment decisions. Keep in mind that the treatment rec-ommendations for these hypothetical scenarios are not necessarily applicable to your personal situation, and I strongly recommend that all aspects of a patient's health be evaluated and considered before pursuing treatment with medications or other modalities. (This com-mentary was originally published in the *NYU Langone Online Journal of Medicine*.)

Consider... a 60-year-old woman, 110 pounds, five feet tall, with no family history or personal history of fracture, no history of smoking or use of steroids. Using the FRAX tool, her 10-year risk of hip fracture is 1.0% and major OP [osteoporosis] fracture is 7.9%. If we made that patient 200 pounds, her risk would be 0.5%. If we gave that same 110-pound patient a history of a parent with an osteoporotic fracture, her risk would rise to 1.9%. Now add to that a personal history of smoking. Her risk rises to 2.85%. Did I mention that she's had IBD (irritable bowel disease) and has been treated over the years with low doses of glucocorticoids? Her risk now rises to 5.9%. Lastly, she drinks every night. Now this patient's risk is 9.0%. But notice how powerful age is as a risk factor: If we made the 60-year-old woman 80 years old, 110 pounds, five feet tall, with no family or personal history of fractures, no history of smoking, and no use of steroids, her 10-year risk of hip fracture would be 10% in 10 years and she would have a 35% chance of the development of any "major osteoporotic" fracture.

The question then becomes, how do numbers translate to treatment? Based on a cost effectiveness analysis, the "magic number" to consider medication is a 3% risk of hip fracture in 10 years or a 20% risk of any other major osteoporotic fracture. For most, the treatment of choice is a bisphosphonate with 1,500 mg of calcium and 1,000 IU of vitamin D and regular weight-bearing exercise.

Note: The FRAX model is frequently updated, so the numbers mentioned in the above example may not match the current model if the same criteria were plugged in.

As mentioned earlier the ten-year probable fracture risk assessment that results from a FRAX calculation should *not* be the only or the main criteria used for prescribing osteoporosis medications. The "magic number" doctors often use (see above) for recommending medications is when, according to the patient's FRAX results, the hip fracture risk is above 3 percent and the risk for other major fractures is above 20 percent. By that measure, all women age seventy who weigh 130 pounds and are five feet five inches tall, and who have normal to borderline osteoporosis (a T-score of –2.5) and no other risk factors would qualify for medication.

Remember: There are a host of individual factors that must be considered before decisions are made regarding a treatment protocol. No *one* measurement should be the determining factor.

The NOGG emphasizes that both the FRAX calculation(s) and the NOGG treatment guidelines should be regarded as information *only*—not as the definitive, final word on treatment options. While FRAX presents useful data, doctors must still make their own assessments of the individuals in their care in order to help them reach decisions about medications and other issues. Simply looking at FRAX or even DXA results and then automatically prescribing osteoporosis drugs is not the equivalent of an assessment. As the International Society for Clinical Densitometry (ISCD) states in its review of the clinical use of fracture risk models, *"[T]here are no published studies showing that any fracture model clearly supersedes a clinician's own judgment."*

Doctors must use their own expertise and experience with a patient rather than rely strictly on a computerized tool. Primary care doctors in particular need to heed this advice because even though FRAX was originally designed for their use they may or may not have expertise in treating osteoporosis. If you are a patient of a physician who is not versed in the complexities of bone health, you may need to press for referrals to specialists and/or insist on additional testing and evaluations (such as those discussed in the next chapter) before making final choices about treatment.

FRAX and DXA Testing: Alone? Together?

If you calculate your fracture risk using the FRAX tool, do you still need a DXA test to determine your BMD? What about the reverse situation: If you've checked your BMD, do you need to bother with FRAX? And is there an alternative to FRAX?

You will probably hear and read conflicting responses to these questions, and different doctors follow different practices. The observations and guidelines below can help clarify several of the issues. Later in the chapter I describe the FORE Fracture Risk Calculator, an alternative tool that I recommend over FRAX.

FRAX + DXA

Some DXA machines are equipped with specialized FRAX software. In such cases, the results from both assessments should be included in the report. Some doctors may also conduct the FRAX assessment during your office visit by utilizing an online program. (*Note:* Only the FRAX tool, not the risk calculator offered through FORE, is currently included for use in some DXA devices.)

FRAX First

Some doctors—and some health services in different parts of the world—recommend checking the FRAX calculations first. Then, depending on the results, a primary care physician may subsequently order DXA testing to assess BMD. The U.S. Preventive Services Task Force, for instance, considers FRAX to be one method for determining whether women under age sixty-five should have a DXA test or not. Although this is the official recommendation from the Task Force, note that patients who have risk factors that are not included in the FRAX model could be falsely assessed as not needing a DXA.

DXA First

A DXA test provides useful data about bone mineral density levels, but as noted throughout this book, BMD is only one of the factors that contribute to fracture risk. That being the case, after a DXA test doctors and/or patients may decide to use FRAX to check other risk factors. It may also be important to look into other lab testing (described in the next chapter). In this way, patients obtain more complete data as to their bone health, which can better inform nutrition, exercise and overall treatment decisions.

FRAX Alone

In a few areas of the world, including some parts of the United States, DXA testing is unavailable, expensive, or hard to access. By contrast, FRAX is free and relatively simple to navigate, so it may be the sole assessment used for some patients. If fracture risks prove high enough, such patients may be prescribed osteoporosis medications solely on the basis of FRAX results.

FRAX Drawbacks

Since its first appearance in 2008 the FRAX tool has evolved, and some problematic elements have been eliminated along the way. The program will continue to be updated. Risk models, however, have inherent limitations, and although FRAX has its strong points, it has weaknesses as well. As stated previously, FRAX is not meant to circumvent the judgment of a doctor who specializes in bone health. And the need for a complete workup on a patient is underscored by the very long list of risk factors for osteoporosis and fractures outlined later in this chapter.

In general terms, the main drawback to FRAX is that it does not take into account all fracture risks or certain variables that affect those risks. Here's what I mean:

- *Fracture history:* FRAX asks if you have *ever* sustained a fracture. Fracturing a bone at the age of twelve after falling hard off a moving bike, for instance, is considerably different from fracturing a bone after a simple fall on grass at the age of fifty. Another question asks whether either parent ever sustained a hip fracture, but doesn't ask how or when. A parent breaking a hip resulting from a head-on car collision at age ninety-five is very different from a parent breaking a hip at age seventy after sustaining only minimal trauma. If you answer yes to the question about your parent breaking a hip, regardless of how it occurred, your probable ten-year fracture risk will be higher.

- *Current smoking:* FRAX assesses for current smoking, but any past history of smoking, which could have resulted in previous bone loss, is not considered.

- *Glucocorticoids:* Variations in risks associated with high or low doses of these medications are not accounted for; clinicians are advised to assume "average" exposure and use their judgment on this point.

- *Secondary osteoporosis:* FRAX accounts for only a very limited number of conditions that contribute to secondary osteoporosis. (A more complete list of the causes of secondary osteoporosis appears later in the chapter.)

o. *Alcohol use:* As with the smoking assessment, FRAX considers only *current* alcohol use and an intake of no more than two or three drinks/day. This can be misleading for many reasons; for example, if you abused alcohol for a period of time at *any* point in your life, it could have resulted in lost bone tissue. Also, many alcoholic beverages contain added sugar. I think a few servings of alcohol each week may be okay for some, but I am opposed to daily consumption for both bone health and overall health.

o *Femoral neck measurement:* FRAX uses *only* the femoral neck BMD. It does not consider BMD measurement of the spine, because when FRAX was developed the data were less clear for the ten-year probability of fracture utilizing measurement of the lumbar spine. And, yes, ignoring spine BMD can lead to an inaccurate risk calculation.

Another drawback to FRAX that cannot be overlooked is that some people will be prescribed medications based on its limited assessment capabilities. It should also be noted that patients who are already taking osteoporosis medications should *not* use FRAX, as they will be unable to get an accurate assessment.

FORE's Fracture Risk Calculator: A FRAX Alternative

FRAX is not the only tool available for estimating fracture risks. The Foundation for Osteoporosis Research and Education (FORE) has developed its own Fracture Risk Calculator (FRC), which can also be found online. To access it, visit the FORE website at www.fore.org or that of its affiliated organization, American Bone Health, at www.americanbonehealth.org.

The FORE calculator essentially aligns with the United States version of FRAX while differing in some important respects. For example, as of late 2012 the FORE calculator for health care professionals considers additional risk factors as well as dosage levels of glucocorticoids. Like FRAX it will continue to be updated. Notably, the FRC also asks for results of bone mineral density measurements of the spine, not just the neck of the femur.

FRC provides users with a graphic representation of risk levels, which can make it easier for patients to see and understand their potential for breaking a bone. An example of an FRC chart is shown in Figure 4.1. First note the three divisions of fracture risk: zero to 10 percent, 10 to 20 percent, and greater than 20 percent. You may recall that these represent low, medium, and high risk, respectively. Next note the dotted line, which represents the average woman's ten-year risk of sustaining any of four types of fracture: hip, shoulder, forearm, or spine. Our sample patient, represented by the dot labeled "Your Risk," is a sixty-two-year-old Caucasian woman. She's five feet five inches tall, weighs 120 pounds, and doesn't smoke. Her ten-year risk for any fracture is 15 percent, which, as you can see, is greater than average (but still in the "medium" range). In addition to what is shown on the graph, FRC also provides information on a patient's ten-year risk of hip fracture. In our sample patient's case, that risk was calculated at 2 percent.

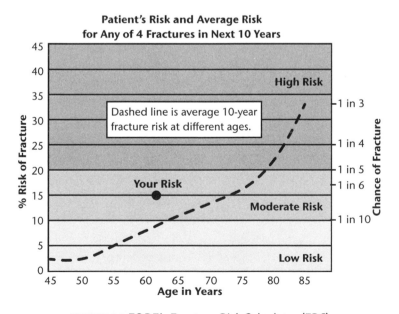

FIGURE 4.1. FORE's Fracture Risk Calculator (FRC)

Risk Factors for Fractures and Osteoporosis

We know a lot about bone development and the factors that impact bone positively and negatively throughout a lifetime. However, we don't know everything there is to know because bone tissue is very complex. Your genetic heritage, of course, has a major impact on the bone mass development that occurs as you grow into adulthood. But nutrition, hormones, health habits, and lifestyle choices also play important roles.

This means that the risks to your bones can be complex and wide-ranging. Some of the well-known factors that influence the probability that you might develop osteoporosis or fracture—for instance, age or gender—were listed in this chapter's discussion on FRAX. Others, however, such as the use of certain medications, and medical conditions that give rise to bone loss, are not generally emphasized during discussions about fracture risks.

> If you have a chronic health condition or are taking any medications, find out whether they could impact your bone health.

The lists below are adapted from those provided by the National Institutes of Health (NIH) and the National Osteoporosis Foundation (NOF). Many of the risks listed are generally accepted as secondary causes for osteoporosis. You can find out more about them by searching online for "NIH-osteoporosis" or by visiting the NOF website.

Conditions Associated with Osteoporosis

- rheumatoid arthritis
- eating disorders, past and present
- malabsorption diseases
- ulcerative colitis
- Crohn's disease
- celiac disease
- depression
- epilepsy
- hyperthyroidism and hypothyroidism
- hypochlorhydria
- breast cancer
- diabetes
- nutritional disorders
- poor health/frailty

- adrenal diseases
- heart disease
- endometriosis
- idiopathic scoliosis
- kidney disease
- hyperparathyroidism

- hyperprolactinemia
- hypogonadism in men or women
- amenorrhea for an extended time
- polycystic ovary syndrome
- premature ovarian failure

Demographics (Not Modifiable)
- Caucasian or Asian ethnicity
- older age
- thinness or small bones in women
- fracture history as an adult, especially over age fifty
- low body weight (less than about 127 pounds)
- primary relatives with osteoporosis
- genetic disorders that weaken the microarchitecture of bone
- early menopause (before age forty-five)

Surgeries
- gastric or intestinal bypass
- hysterectomy with ovary removal
- thyroidectomy

Lifestyle (Past and Present—Modifiable If Present)
Note that if any of these were problems in the past, the bones may have suffered either from the failure to build a good bank account or even possibly from bone loss.
- cigarette smoking
- daily alcohol consumption
- use of illicit drugs (e.g., cocaine)
- heavy caffeine intake (generally listed by medical papers as over three servings per day; however, I recommend no more than one serving each day, and ideally none)
- excessive dieting

o diet high in sugar and other junk food

o daily use of soft drinks

o acidic diet—high in meat, sugar, and processed carbohydrates

o high salt intake

o low or excessive protein intake

o chronic antacid use

o vitamin D deficiency

o low long-term calcium intake

o low long-term magnesium intake

o inadequate exercise

o excessive exercise, leading to lowered body fat and amenorrhea

Medications (Past and Present Use)

o proton pump inhibitors (PPIs; e.g., Nexium, Prevacid, Prilosec)

o aluminum-containing antacids

o some antiseizure medicines (e.g., Dilantin, phenobarbital)

o SSRIs (antidepressants)

o some immunosuppressive drugs (e.g., cyclosporine A, tacrolimus/FK506)

o methotrexate

o anticonvulsants

o lithium

o loop diuretics

o aromatase inhibitors (e.g., Arimidex, Aromasin, Femara)

o heparin

o antibiotics (long-term use)

o Depo-Provera

o gonadotropin releasing hormone (GnRH; e.g., Lupron, Zoladex)

o some cancer chemotherapeutic drugs

o tamoxifen (premenopausal use)

o thiazolidinediones (e.g., Actos, Avandia)

o excess thyroid hormone

o corticosteroids (long-term use; see below)

Steroid medications (corticosteroids), one of the most frequently prescribed medications, can have a major impact on bone health. The American College of Rheumatology has estimated that 20 percent of all osteoporosis in the United States is due to use of corticosteroid medications. There are over twenty medications in the category of corticosteroids; three of the more commonly prescribed are prednisone, cortisone, and hydrocortisone. Long-term (six months) chronic use of inhaled corticosteroids, to treat asthma or other lung conditions, has been associated with increased fractures and bone loss.

The above is just a partial list of medications that can impact bone health. More medications will likely be added to this list. For more information about this topic, visit the National Osteoporosis Foundation website (www.nof.org).

Responding to Risk

The point of using tools such as FRAX and the FORE Fracture Risk Calculator is not to develop a definitive diagnosis. Rather, they—and the above risk factor lists—are designed to provide additional information that you and your physician need to consider if you are to give your bones the best care possible.

Some risk factors, of course, are beyond your control—for instance, genetics and gender. In addition, even if you don't smoke cigarettes or drink heavily today, if you smoked or drank for a period of time in your earlier years, it is possible that those behaviors could have resulted in bone loss. Likewise, if you had poor eating habits as a teenager and thus did not get enough calcium, you may not have gained an optimal peak bone mass to begin with. That said, the presence of risk factors—current or past—that are beyond your control does not mean that you cannot reduce your exposure to fracture risk. You can quit smoking, decrease salt and sugar intake, boost your exercise program, and improve your balance, for example.

The main thing to remember is this: Make sure you are not losing bone presently. Any occurrence of ongoing bone loss can only be determined through good detective work by your doctor, which should include bone density screening, a thorough review of your medical history, and appropriate lab testing. In the next chapter you'll learn some of the detective's strategies for assessing health history and using different lab tests to pinpoint the issues that affect a person's bone health.

 KEY POINTS FROM CHAPTER 4

- It is important to know your personal risk factors for osteoporosis.

- The FRAX tool can help you determine your probable ten-year fracture risk.

- The FRAX tool is *only one* piece of information regarding your bone health.

- The FRAX tool can over- or underestimate your ten-year fracture risk.

- When compared to the FRAX tool, the FORE Fracture Risk Calculator (FRC) includes additional risk factors in its calculations.

- You can use both tools (FRAX and FRC) online without having results from a bone density test.

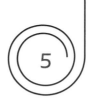

Beyond Bone Density Testing: What's *Really* Going On in Your Body?

Bone is typically silent. It rarely announces problems through symptoms like the aches that turn up with a sore muscle or the fatigue and fever that often accompany the flu. To discover the true condition of your bones, it takes a little detective work.

Certainly, bone density testing can be a valuable part of the investigative process because it supplies an important measurement. And a FRAX assessment offers a numerical estimate of future fracture risk. These two pieces of data, however, do not add up to the total sum of information needed to understand the state of your bone health. They do not answer a fundamental question: Why? If it has been determined that you are losing bone, or if you are fracturing bones, it is crucial for you and your doctor to know *why*, if at all possible. This essential question needs to be answered before any treatment program begins.

As you learned in Chapter 1, bone loss may be related to advancing age and/or estrogen depletion, among other causes. Or perhaps you never built up an adequate supply of bone in your early years, so you are more susceptible to osteoporosis or fractures later in life. Or maybe something else is going on. You may not be absorbing calcium or other bone nutrients. It's possible that a smoking habit or a digestive problem could be affecting your skeletal structure. Then again, there might be another disease process at work that is depleting the bones and producing a troublesome bone density reading. To tease out the reasons why you may be losing bone or fracturing, your health-care provider should do a thorough medical assessment, including diagnostic lab tests and a full review of your health history.

In this chapter you will be introduced to some of the lab tests that may be ordered in medical assessments of osteoporosis or low bone density. The chapter also offers an overview of the key issues in your past and present health history that could be affecting your current bone health. The goal here is not to turn you into a medical expert or to promote unnecessary lab tests. Rather, it is to give you a basic understanding of the investigative work that needs to be done to discover the source of your bone health problems, if possible. The first step is to recognize that it's important to go deeper than surface assessments and closely examine the overall condition of your body.

Why It's Important to Dig Deep

As stated earlier, bone is silent, and osteoporosis is referred to as a silent disease (which seems to be the case until you fracture a bone). Yet bone is also complex, and just as any other major medical condition can be complicated, so, too, can health problems that involve the bones.

Bone's complexity is not always addressed in medical consultations during which patients learn the results of a bone density test and receive prescriptions for medications. A hurried approach to patient care can short-circuit the important process of fully analyzing a person's health. Furthermore, the tendency in conventional Western medicine to treat symptoms rather than causes can lead to misdiagnoses or missed cues that may point to problems beyond a low bone density reading.

When diagnosing bone problems, it is important to remember that there are several types of osteoporosis (as explained in Chapter 1). To recap, these include:

- o primary osteoporosis, which is largely attributable to aging and/or postmenopausal estrogen loss (note, however, that I do not subscribe to the notion that bone loss is *inevitable* with aging or during menopause) o idiopathic osteoporosis, in which the cause cannot be determined

o secondary osteoporosis, which stems from diseases, conditions, medications, or lifestyle issues that are not found in the other osteoporosis categories

Secondary osteoporosis (see risk factor list in Chapter 4) can arise from a host of causes ranging from the use of steroids or proton pump inhibitors, to the lack of vitamin D, to thyroid problems or gastrointestinal issues. By conducting lab tests, doctors are better able to identify or rule out possible secondary causes of a patient's osteoporosis and determine whether she or he is *currently* losing bone. For example, if you had an eating disorder twenty years ago and you lost bone back then, and now you eat a healthy diet, you may not be losing bone now. (However, you could still have osteoporosis today because of the anorexia years earlier.)

Not every patient, of course, needs a full complement of laboratory tests. Generally, doctors tend to order lab tests on the basis of how significant the osteoporosis is, or if it is known that bone loss has occurred. Those criteria, however, are not foolproof, because some doctors may start treatment without first delving into the possible causes of a patient's bone-health problems. For certain patients, an undetected medical condition might be the culprit, but that possibility can be overlooked if doctors reach for the prescription pad before conducting further lab tests and doing a dietary analysis. When dealing with bone health, therefore, it is important for doctors and patients to keep an open mind about causal factors.

Stephen's case, described below, dramatically illustrates the importance of remaining open to diagnostic clues rather than jumping to conclusions about bone conditions or hastily prescribing osteoporosis drugs.

 ### *Is There an Underlying Reason for Osteoporosis? Stephen's Story*

Stephen's medium build and the lack of fractures in his health history did not seem to indicate someone who could receive a diagnosis of osteoporosis at age forty-seven. But as I reviewed his

(cont'd.)

medical information, I began to question that assumption, and I decided to order lab tests. The test results revealed that Stephen had primary hyperparathyroidism. His previous doctors had not ordered the test that would divulge his condition; instead, he was offered the osteoporosis drug Fosamax right off the bat, without any further evaluation.

If Stephen had taken the recommended medication, his parathyroid tumor would have continued to be a problem, because the doctor would not have treated the actual cause of his bone loss—that is, the hyperparathyroidism, which is considered one of the secondary conditions that give rise to bone loss and, eventually, osteoporosis. Stephen would have continued to lose bone, and his parathyroid tumor may have worsened. By taking the time to accurately assess Stephen's case, which included an order for lab tests to uncover the reasons for his bone loss, I was able to educate him about the problem and refer him for proper treatment. In this case, treatment involved a fairly simple surgical procedure to remove the problematic parathyroid gland.

Once a secondary condition such as hyperparathyroidism is addressed, bone density levels can improve. That turned out to be the case for Stephen: Two years after surgery his bone density had increased by 10 percent. Remember, osteoporosis treatments will be ineffective if a secondary medical condition that is causing bone loss is not resolved first.

The Story of Your Bones: A Personal Health History

Upon arriving at a doctor's office, the first thing patients typically do is fill out an intake form, answering questions about their medical history quickly and from memory. Then, because of the rushed pace of many health consultations, physicians may have little opportunity to focus on the forms or carefully analyze a patient's history.

These brief interactions can prevent both patient and physician from digging into a gold mine of information that may lead to more accurate diagnostic and treatment decisions. With the complex issue of bone health—which is impacted by so many different factors over the course of decades in a person's life—it is crucial to conduct an in-depth review of a patient's health background.

Doctors would not quarrel with the idea that knowing a patient's medical history helps them arrive at a diagnosis in the majority of cases. A study published in the *Archives of Internal Medicine* confirms this fact. Researchers reported that patients' medical history "emerged as the key element in formulating correct diagnosis" of medical conditions. Some health practitioners estimate that as much as 80 percent of a diagnosis comes from taking a good health history and a full assessment of the patient's symptoms.

In my own practice, it takes one to two hours to discuss the extensive questionnaire my patients receive, which covers not only their past medical history but also other factors that might impact their bones—such as balance problems, sleeping patterns, diet, and gastrointestinal health issues. This discussion serves several purposes. For one, until I go over the patient's health history, I won't know which lab tests to order as part of the process to help determine if active bone loss may be occurring and, if so, its potential causes. In addition, the lengthy consultation allows time to truly hear about what has happened or is happening in patients' lives that could explain the condition of their current bone health. I also believe the adage that has circulated among health-care practitioners for many years: *Your patients will tell you the diagnosis if you listen to them.*

Does Your Doctor Listen to You?

A standard question I pose to my patients is this: "Does your doctor listen to you?" I also ask them to think about how comfortable they feel with their doctors or other health-care practitioners they may be working with. People who respond positively have a better chance of partnering with their physicians to get to the bottom of their bone-health problems and other conditions. People who respond negatively, by contrast, may need to search for another physician or possibly consult with other practitioners who can answer their questions. Unfortunately, our current managed health care system prevents many doctors from fully delving into a patient's medical and family history in order to discover the full range of issues that impact the bones. And even the most sensitive doctors may lack the appropriate expertise to answer all of your questions, so they might have to refer you to a bone specialist, a nutritionist, or other practitioners. Then, however, another problem arises, because when several specialists are involved in a case, they do not generally consult with each other, so no single practitioner has a complete view of a patient's health.

All of this means that patients have to gather their personal information and investigate some questions on their own. For instance, if a parent broke a hip, it's important to consider how and when it happened. Was it a low-trauma fracture at midlife? Or a break caused by a car crash at a younger age? By the same token, before simply accepting a prescription for osteoporosis medications based on a cursory examination, patients can ask about other lab tests that might be appropriate for them (as discussed later in this chapter).

If you have a positive relationship with your health-care practitioners, use the information in this book to alert them to the issues and questions that concern you so they can think things through on your behalf—and together you can arrive at the best treatment decisions.

Your Health History: Questions to Consider

Medical history forms and the FRAX tool offer a fundamental set of questions commonly used to evaluate bone health and fracture risk. Some of the questions concern basic topics such as family/personal history of broken bones and tobacco/alcohol use. These forms and the FRAX questionnaire are easily found on the Internet. The U.S. Surgeon General's office offers a free online tool called "My Family Health Portrait," which enables users to address a number of questions about medical conditions that affect immediate and extended family members. In addition, the National Osteoporosis Foundation provides an online form called "My Bone History," which, although not extensive, does give patients a simple format for tracking BMD tests and other related bone information, including medications and supplements. This tool is especially handy for doctor visits and health care consultations. You can also review the list of risk factors for osteoporosis that is included in Chapter 4. Finally, you can download the questionnaire used by my patients by visiting www.LaniSimpson.com.

Each of these resources can help you examine your personal health history and the bone-health issues that you may need to bring to the attention of your doctor. As you begin to document your medical history, some of the main questions you should consider include the following:

- o *Family history of broken bones?* Remember, genetics is one of the key factors that affect fracture risk. Gather as much information as you can about broken bones experienced by either of your parents as well as grandparents and siblings. When a significant number of fractures are found in an extended family group, it's possible that members of the family have an inherited weakness. Information on parents is particularly important; it is known that if parents fracture a hip, it increases the likelihood that their children will incur the same fate. However, keep the fractures in perspective. If your mother broke her hip falling down stairs at the age of ninety-eight, that is different from stumbling and breaking a hip at the age of eighty.

- o *Personal history of fractures?* If you have fractured a bone, you may be at risk of fracturing again. It depends on when, where, and how the bone break occurred. Document your fractures with as much detail as possible. If you fractured a bone falling off of a bike at forty miles per hour at age sixteen, that is different than falling at age forty-five and fracturing a wrist.

- o *Balance problems?* Balance problems can lead to falls, and falls can lead to fractures, so this issue needs to be included in your health history. Too often, patients fail to discuss balance problems with their doctors. Because fall prevention is critical to avoiding fractures, make sure you get any balance issues evaluated. Commonly, an inner ear problem can cause vertigo, while a drop in blood pressure can create dizziness when a person quickly stands up from a sitting position. Many other potentially harmful conditions can also cause dizziness or vertigo. Do not ignore this symptom!

○ *Are your muscles in good shape?* As mentioned earlier, sarcopenia (muscle wasting) is common in elderly people with osteoporosis. You will reduce fractures by keeping muscles in shape in terms of both strength and flexibility (a topic you will learn more about in Chapter 11).

○ *Alcohol use and smoking?* It is easy to underestimate one's amount and frequency of alcohol and tobacco consumption, but accuracy matters because both substances have a detrimental effect on bones. The FRAX tool takes into account only current use of cigarettes and alcohol, but past smoking or drinking can also negatively impact bone. Make certain, then, to include previous smoking and drinking habits in your personal health history. The same goes for illicit drug use, whether past or present. It should be considered as part of your personal health history.

○ *Height loss?* Height loss can be an indication of skeletal problems. As mentioned in Chapter 1, to ensure consistent height measurements it is crucial to measure your height at roughly the same time each day using an accurate technique. The combination height/weight scale commonly found in doctor's offices is not always reliable. A simple measuring tape attached to the side of a doorway works fine. Just be sure to stand erect with your back against the tape. Then have a family member or friend place something flat, such as a clipboard, on top of your head, and make a pencil mark on the tape to record your height.

○ *Secondary osteoporosis?* The FRAX assessment includes a question on some of the risk factors associated with secondary osteoporosis. Some of these factors are addressed in more detail in this chapter's sections on lab tests.

○ *Gastrointestinal health/nutrition issues?* Even though the status of a person's diet and gastrointestinal health has a great influence on the condition of their bones, few doctors understand or examine these issues in-depth. At the very least, keeping a diary for seven days of everything you eat and noting any gastrointestinal distress during that week can provide valuable insight into these important issues. It is also helpful for you to make note of any other times you may have experienced gastrointestinal problems. (Chapters 9 and 10 discuss the links between nutrition, digestion, and bones in more detail.)

o *Irregular sleeping patterns?* The body repairs itself during sleep, and the length and quality of your sleep affects your bone health. As people age, a good night's sleep is often more difficult to achieve—but that does not mean you should ignore sleep deprivation or write it off as something that just happens as you get older. Keep a sleep diary showing the times when you go to bed and awaken. The following questions will help you evaluate your sleeping patterns: In general, are you getting enough sleep at night? How many hours of sleep do you get each night? How long does it take for you to fall asleep? What time do you go to bed? What activities do you engage in prior to bedtime? Do you wake up with an alarm clock or without one? Do you wake up tired? If you have sleeping difficulties, how long has this been the case? Are you taking anything to induce sleep? Is your sleep interrupted, and if it is, what causes the interruption? Do pets wake you up, or is something else causing your sleep loss? Include your answers to these questions in your health history, and begin taking a few simple steps to improve your sleep if you're having difficulties. For example, shut off electronics two hours before bed, keep the bedroom cool at night, use light-blocking curtains to help keep the bedroom dark while you're in bed, and go to bed and rise at the same times every day.

Lose Sleep, Lose Bone?

One study published in the journal *Experimental Biology and Medicine* showed a decrease in bone density in sleep-deprived rats. Abnormalities were found in bone and bone marrow in the animals who experienced a chronic lack of sleep. Getting enough rest is restorative and important to staying healthy—and that applies to bone health, as well.

o *Emotional health?* Stress, including emotional upheavals, takes a toll on skeletal remodeling by increasing inflammation. Excessive stress releases the hormone cortisol. The right amount of cortisol is healthy and necessary for the body, but excess cortisol can lead to bone loss. Cortisol levels can be checked using urine, blood, or saliva tests.

o *Female health issues?* Pregnancies, contraceptive use, and menopause are all issues that women need to think about when it comes to their bone health, because all of them affect bone mineral density and fracture risk. Be sure your doctor is aware of all aspects of your gynecological health, past and present. For instance, if your menstrual cycle started at age eighteen, it could result in a lower peak bone mass at the end of your twenties. Or if you missed menstrual cycles regularly during your menstru- ating years, it could explain low bone mass later in life. Also, as you've read throughout this book, the loss of estrogen during menopause can lead to a significant decrease in BMD. If you are about to enter menopause, it is crucial to recognize the impact of this life passage on your bones. Whether you are pre- or post- menopausal, you can always take steps to improve your bone health through diet, exercise, and supplements.

o *Medications?* The medications listed in Chapter 4 are known to be possible contributors to bone loss; be sure to discuss with your doctor whether any of them may be contributing to bone-related problems for you. Remember, too, that harmful drug interactions can be life threatening, so it is important to keep the list of the medications you're taking up-to-date and to consult with your physician, pharmacist, and any others on your health team to stay aware of potential problems. Do not stop taking your medications after simply reading the list in Chap- ter 4. Always consult with your doctor. Stopping medications abruptly can result in a rebound effect that is very unpleasant and in some cases dangerous.

o *Supplements?* Besides recording your use of medications, it's also important to include in your health history the intake of any vitamin supplements or herbs. Document any adverse reac- tions you have experienced. Some herbs may interfere with the effectiveness of certain medications, so it is important to provide information on your use of herbs and supplements to the health professionals who care for you.

To maximize your effectiveness as your own health advocate, keep notes on doctor visits and on your health history. Be sure to get personal copies of lab reports, X-rays, diagnostic pages from DXA tests, and any other paperwork related to your care. I often advise my patients to organize their records and health history in a three-ring binder so it's easy to review. If and when electronic medical records become the norm, you may not wish to maintain paper records. Certain software and mobile apps can also work if you prefer digital records to a binder full of paper. Regardless of whether or not medical information is in digital form, it's still up to you to keep track of your own health care needs and experiences. Use whatever form of record keeping works best for you—and remember, no one else knows your body better than you do.

Examining Bone Health Histories: Looking Past the Obvious

Since the World Health Organization established parameters in the 1990s for the diagnosis of osteoporosis based on BMD readings and T-scores, the evaluation of bone health has become more standardized. The downside of this standardization, however, is that it can lead health-care practitioners to view patients' health through the one-dimensional lens of DXA tests or to settle on a diagnosis before fully examining an individual's medical history. Remember, bone-health issues are complex! So it is important for doctors to avoid jumping to conclusions or making surface judgments about a patient's condition, as the following example shows:

> *A Convergence of Factors: Caroline's Story*
> *Several issues seemed to indicate that fifty-seven-year-old Caroline was a prime candidate for bone problems. Not only was she postmenopausal, but her dentist had told her that she was losing bone in her jaw. In addition, in the course of a hip replacement Caroline's surgeon noted that she had "soft bones." Her primary doctor ordered a bone density test, which came back as a –1.8 in the spine and –1.2 in the hip. At that time she*
> (cont'd.)

was diagnosed with osteopenia. Finally, a bone marker test was very high, indicating she might be losing bone.

In reviewing all of these factors, I first asked that Caroline check with the dentist to find out whether she was losing bone throughout the jaw, or if instead the bone loss might be due to infection, in which case it would be localized to one specific area. As it turned out, the jawbone loss was limited to an area of infection, which meant that it did not suggest pervasive bone-health problems. Next, a follow-up bone marker test revealed that Caroline's first test was incorrect; in fact, results from the new test showed that she was well within the normal range. Finally, when Caroline's surgeon and others use a vague description like "soft bone," they are not usually referring to osteoporotic bone, which is better described as "brittle." The term "soft bone" led me to question whether Caroline had some other problem, such as a vitamin D deficiency or another condition that might be inhibiting her absorption of calcium. Indeed, testing proved that Caroline's vitamin D levels were very low.

Among other steps to improve her bone health, Caroline increased her intake of vitamin D. Overall, however, her health was quite good. She had strong muscles and had never fractured a bone, and her need of a hip replacement had been due to injuries sustained in a car accident. Caroline's story underscores the importance of closely examining lab reports and professional opinions before making a final judgment on a diagnosis or treatment plan.

Do You Need Lab Tests?

When it comes to bone conditions, how do doctors decide which patients need lab tests? And when should you, as a patient, ask for more tests?

Obviously, the answers to these questions depend on a myriad of individual factors ranging from age and gender to symptoms and family history, among others. For many doctors, your BMD reading from a DXA test and/or your degree of fracture risk as measured by the FRAX questionnaire will be used to gauge whether lab tests are needed.

Typically, lab tests are ordered for the following groups of people:

o patients who are actively losing bone (as indicated either by two accurately assessed DXA tests usually two-plus years apart, or by previous lab tests that were positive for potential bone loss, such as bone markers or thyroid tests—see below)

o patients experiencing low-trauma, fragility fractures (and, sometimes, those over age fifty experiencing any type of fracture)

o patients with osteoporosis (as determined by their bone mineral density readings and T-scores)

o patients who have chronic digestive symptoms or other health issues that might result in secondary bone loss

Are you really losing bone? The results from lab work as well as DXA scans can help determine the answer to that question. For instance, a lab test can reveal if conditions such as kidney disease or thyroid problems are contributing to bone loss. When it comes to BMD testing, however, what often happens is that a patient gets *one* DXA scan that shows low bone density or even osteoporosis, and many doctors assume the patient is currently, actively losing bone. Such an assumption is similar to looking at one monthly bank statement from a business and concluding that the company is losing money. Obviously, a minimum of several bank statements must be compared—and other factors taken into account—before drawing any kind of conclusion about a company's profit and loss.

Similarly, patients need at least *two* DXA tests before anyone can begin to make judgments about the gain or loss of bone mineral density. (And remember, those tests must be conducted properly; see Chapter 2.) As explained previously, a small person or someone who did not build up their bones in early life will most likely start off with a baseline BMD that is in the low range. Just because that baseline is low, however, does not mean the person's BMD is decreasing. This issue becomes important because it impacts treatment decisions. In addition, a patient with active bone loss, as opposed to stable bone, is the more likely candidate for extensive lab testing. What is the difference between the two states?

o *Active bone loss* means bone loss is likely occurring *presently,* based on a comparison between the results of at least *two* accurate bone density exams and/or through lab work following a thorough case history.

o *Stable bone* means no bone loss is likely occurring presently— even though the patient may have low bone density or osteoporosis. Bone loss may have occurred in the *past,* or the patient might be a small person to begin with. As with active bone loss, bone stability is determined by comparing the results of two accurate bone density exams and/or through lab work that is ordered after a thorough case history assessment.

Lab Tests: Filling In Your Bone-Health Picture

Medical laboratory tests provide measurements of bodily functions that can supplement data from DXA tests, FRAX calculations, and your personal risk profile, health history, and dietary analysis. Taken together, all of this information creates a well-rounded assessment of your bone health that can be used in making decisions about treatment. For some of my patients, it's helpful for them to think of these various types of medical information as wedges in a pie chart—BMD readings form one slice, FRAX calculations form a second, lab results a third, lifestyle a fourth, and so on.

When it comes to bone health, laboratory tests are primarily used to determine if secondary causes could be the reason for a low bone density reading, a fracture, or a diagnosis of osteoporosis. To discover these causes, doctors may order a set of basic lab tests as well as other, specific tests for certain conditions and diseases associated with osteoporosis. Both basic and some of the more commonly ordered specific tests are described below.

Though every case of osteoporosis is unique, certain lab tests are appropriate for a broad range of patients. In my practice, the assessment of a patient's health history influences the tests that I decide to order. The patient's BMD reading, of course, plays a part as well. Someone with a T-score of –2.0 who is fit and has no significant risk factors other than the low bone density reading will not require the extensive testing of someone with a clear diagnosis of osteoporosis and/or a significant fracture risk.

This section discusses some of the most important lab tests related to bone health. (There are numerous other tests as well, which only underscores the fact that bone health is a complex issue that should be analyzed from many angles.) All of the tests listed here can reveal useful information. To simplify matters, I have broken them down into two lists: basic tests, and those warranted based on the patient's history and/or bone density report. Most of the tests involve the use of blood (sometimes labeled as tests for levels of "serum"—a term which, essentially, refers to a component of blood). Urine tests are noted as such.

Note: Medications can impact laboratory findings. If you have an abnormal test, check to see if any of your medications are known to affect lab results or contribute to bone loss. In addition, keep in mind that lab results can also be incorrect and often need to be repeated. Sometimes I will send a patient to an entirely different lab group for a second round of tests if I question the findings.

Basic Lab Tests

1. CBC (complete blood count)
2. Comprehensive blood chemistry panel
3. Vitamin D (25-hydroxyvitamin D or 25(OH)D)
4. TSH (thyroid function)

Additional Lab Tests (Ordering Depends on Individual Case History)

5. PTH-intact (parathyroid function)
6. Calcium (serum calcium and ionized calcium)
7. 24-hour urine test (calcium and creatinine)
8. GFR (glomerular filtration rate)
9. Creatinine (CCr or CrCl)
10. Magnesium RBC (this is the best of the magnesium tests to order)
11. Phosphorus

12. Celiac profile

13. Hormone tests for men and women (estradiol, testosterone, DHEA, progesterone)

14. Cortisol

15. Homocysteine

16. HS-CRP (high-sensitivity C-reactive protein)

17. Bone markers

18. Erythrocyte sedimentation rate (ESR)

19. Prolactin

20. Protein electrophoresis (to rule out multiple myeloma)

21. Calcitriol (1,25-dihydroxyvitamin D or 1,25(OH)2D)

22. Lipid peroxides and 8OH2dG

Keep in mind that an astute clinician will make note of a lab test that is within normal limits yet might still be a problem. Some of the tests where the low end of a normal reading may point to a potential problem include blood results for calcium, protein, and magnesium. A high end of normal reading for calcium and parathyroid hormone may also point to an underlying problem. You will learn more about this in Chapter 8, in the section on calcium-regulating hormones.

Here are brief descriptions of each of the lab tests listed above:

1. CBC (Complete Blood Count)

The CBC includes eighteen or more tests. It is a broad screening of blood to determine an individual's general health status. A wide range of diseases or conditions can be discovered with a CBC, including anemia (caused by deficiencies in iron or vitamin B-12) and other conditions that can cause bone loss.

2. Comprehensive Blood Chemistry Panel

Includes fourteen or more tests and provides a general look at how body systems and organs are functioning, including the liver and kidneys. Specific tests in this panel that can point to bone problems include those that check levels of calcium, protein, phosphorus, sodium, and blood sugar.

3. Vitamin D (25-Hydroxyvitamin D or 25(OH)D)

Vitamin D plays a crucial role in calcium absorption. A low vitamin D test can indicate a vitamin D deficiency and possibly a calcium deficiency. There are two vitamin D tests. Make sure you get the assessment for 25(OH)D. A different vitamin D test—1,25(OH)D—is only ordered for specific diagnostic purposes (see #21 below).

4. TSH (Thyroid Stimulating Hormone)

TSH is the standard test to check for hypo- or hyperthyroidism, either of which can result in bone loss if not treated appropriately. Other thyroid tests that might be ordered when thyroid disease is suspected include: thyroid antibody tests, free T3, free T4, total T3 and T4, reverse T3, and ferritin. When it comes to diagnosing hypothyroidism, sometimes the results can be within normal limits, yet the patient still shows multiple symptoms. See Chapter 8. Testing levels of the adrenal hormones DHEA and cortisol might also be helpful (see #13 and #14).

5. PTH-Intact (Parathyroid Function)

The parathyroid glands are pivotal for bone health. (In Chapter 8 you will learn about the importance of these four tiny glands located in the neck just behind the thyroid gland.) Hyperparathyroidism (excessive parathyroid hormone secretion) can result in bone loss. This condition should be checked in anyone diagnosed with osteoporosis. The PTH-intact test must be ordered with serum calcium, because they need to be analyzed together. Some labs (e.g., Quest Diagnostics) freeze the PTH specimen, which yields more accurate results.

6. Calcium Tests

There are two different tests to check calcium in the blood: serum calcium and ionized calcium.

- *Serum calcium* is the total calcium found in a blood sample; it may be listed on reports as "serum calcium," "calcium total," or simply "calcium." The test for serum calcium is included in blood chemistry panels, but it can also be ordered separately.
- *Ionized calcium* is freely floating in the blood, i.e., not bound to protein.

Low serum or ionized calcium points to possible calcium deficiency, malabsorption, or vitamin D deficiency. Elevated calcium or ionized calcium can point to primary hyperparathyroidism, bone cancer, or other conditions.

7. 24-Hour Urine Calcium Excretion Test

Hypercalciuria, or excessive urinary calcium excretion, occurs in about 5 to 10 percent of the population. Depending on the diagnostic tests requested for an individual, the twenty-four-hour urine test can also include testing for sodium excretion or a calcium/creatinine ratio, which can also point to potential bone loss. Preparing for this test is important, so follow all directions from your doctor and from the lab. It is often recommended that you stop all calcium supplements prior to the test, and that you refrain from heavy exercise the day before and the day of testing. This test can easily be incorrect or misleading. It is very important that your doctor be familiar with the test, and it is also important that she retest you, if necessary.

8. Glomerular Filtration Rate (GFR)

Glomerular filtration rate (GFR) describes the flow rate of filtered fluid through the kidney. A low filtration rate indicates poor kidney function. Poor kidney function can result in excess calcium loss in the urine, resulting in bone loss.

9. Creatinine (CCr or CrCl)

The creatinine clearance rate is a useful measure for approximating the GFR (see #8). The results of the GFR and CCr tests are important in assessing the excretory function of the kidneys.

10. Magnesium RBC (Red Blood Cell)

Low magnesium intake, over time, can result in low calcium and potassium levels. Magnesium can be checked in the blood to help diagnose problems with calcium, potassium, phosphorus levels, and/or parathyroid hormone. The best blood test is the magnesium RBC, not simply magnesium. See Chapter 10 for more information on this very important mineral. Low persistent magnesium over time can cause low calcium and potassium levels.

11. Phosphorus

Phosphorus tests are most often ordered along with other tests, such as those for calcium, parathyroid hormone (PTH), and/or vitamin D, to help diagnose and/or monitor treatment of various conditions, including parathyroid disease, gastrointestinal disorders, and kidney disease. It is important that this nutrient be balanced with calcium. See Chapter 10 for more details.

12. Celiac Profile

Celiac disease (CD; gluten intolerance) is a cause of secondary osteoporosis. Over time, this condition results in bone loss due to malabsorption of nutrients. CD is an autoimmune disease. Following are the most important celiac tests:

- antigliadin antibodies—IgG and IgA
- antitissue trans-glutaminase antibody—tTG
- immunoglobulin A (serum total IgA)

Sometimes these tests fail to detect celiac disease. A biopsy of the small intestine by means of an endoscopy is more accurate. However, eliminating gluten can also help diagnose CD.

13. Hormone Tests for Men and Women

Hormonal balance is a key component of building and maintaining healthy bone. These tests include estradiol, estriol, total estrogen, testosterone (free and total), DHEAs, and progesterone. Additional pituitary tests include follicle-stimulating hormone, luteinizing hormone, and prolactin. Women, especially just before and after menopause, typically lose bone due to declining estrogen levels. Testing methods for hormones include serum (blood), saliva, and urine. You will read more about the importance of hormones in Chapter 8. For a list of specialty labs that offer saliva, stool and urine testing, see Resources.

14. Cortisol

A low blood cortisol level can indicate adrenal insufficiency or rare diseases of the adrenal glands, such as Cushing's disease or Addison's disease. Some doctors may order urinary and saliva cortisol. I prefer saliva testing that includes cortisol output four times in one day rather than a single test, especially if I suspect adrenal fatigue. This will give a map of whether cortisol is elevated or depleted at certain times of the day. A balanced nutritional program can support adrenals. See Chapter 8 on hormones for more information.

Blood cortisol is also used to help diagnose adrenal insufficiency and Addison's disease, a condition in which the adrenal glands do not function properly, or Cushing's syndrome, a group of signs and symptoms associated with excess cortisol.

15. Homocysteine

An elevated level of the amino acid homocysteine has been associated with osteoporosis, heart disease, and dementia. Elevated levels may also indicate deficiency of vitamin B-12 or folate (another B vitamin) or malnutrition. See Chapter 10 for more information on the B vitamins and bone health.

16. HS-CRP (High-Sensitivity C-Reactive Protein)

This test serves as a generalized marker of inflammation that is primarily associated with heart disease. Higher circulating levels of CRP have been linked to lower bone density in some studies. Inflammation is discussed in Chapters 9 and 10.

17. Bone Markers

Bone marker tests assess different aspects of bone remodeling, which occurs in a cycle of resorption and bone formation (see Chapter 1). They can provide diagnostic information about bone loss and bone pathology. They are also useful for monitoring treatment, whether it involves osteoporosis medications or changes in diet, exercise, and supplementation. In the medical community, some controversy exists over the use of bone markers. Nonetheless, bone markers are valuable when they are utilized correctly. Make sure your bone specialist is familiar with these tests. Below are the names of some of the more commonly ordered bone marker tests.

Bone Formation Markers
- o osteocalcin
- o bone-specific alkaline phosphatase
- o P1NP (procollagen type 1 N-terminal propeptide)

Bone Resorption Markers (Urine Tests)

- NTx (collagen type 1 cross-linked N-telopeptide, serum or urine)
- CTx (collagen type 1 cross-linked C-telopeptide, serum or urine)
- DPD (deoxypyridinoline cross links, urine. Not recommended at this time; it is less accurate than other bone marker tests)

18. Erythrocyte Sedimentation Rate (ESR)

ESR is an inexpensive, nonspecific test. ESR may be elevated when a patient has an acute or chronic inflammatory condition. Some of the conditions that could underlie an elevated ESR include rheumatoid arthritis, multiple myeloma (a type of bone cancer), and autoimmune diseases.

19. Prolactin

Prolactin is a hormone that is normally high in women during pregnancy, just after childbirth, and throughout nursing. It stimulates milk to be released from the breasts. Either men or women can have a pituitary tumor (usually benign) that increases the blood level of this hormone, which can result in bone loss.

20. Protein Electrophoresis

Used to identify multiple myeloma (a type of bone cancer), this test is ordered in some cases of osteoporosis, especially advanced cases.

21. 1,25-Dihydroxyvitamin D (Calcitriol)

The test for calcitriol may be ordered when calcium is elevated, which can point to parathyroid disease. The final conversion of vitamin D to its hormone form (calcitriol) occurs in the kidney. This test is often called for when kidney disease is suspected. It is not to be confused with the assessment for vitamin D-3 levels—that is, the 25-hydroxyvitamin D (test #3, above). See Chapter 8 for more on this hormone.

22. Lipid Peroxides (Serum) and 8OH2dG (Urine)

These tests evaluate oxidative stress. They are useful for guiding therapy and may be retested in that context.

Quick Reference for Lab Tests

The table below, adapted from a chart created by the Cleveland Clinic, provides a quick reference for checking the names of tests that might be ordered to confirm or eliminate the existence of certain diseases or health problems that could contribute to bone loss or osteoporosis. In medical terms, these health issues are often labeled "comorbidities"—that is, they coexist simultaneously alongside other conditions or diseases. As you will see, some of the tests listed in this table are among those listed above.

Table 5.1. Selected Laboratory Tests for Specific Conditions that Contribute to Osteoporosis

Condition	Appropriate Tests
Acromegaly	Serum IGF-1
Addison's disease	ACTH stimulation test
Cushing's syndrome	24-hour free urinary cortisol; dexamethasone suppression test
Hemochromatosis	Serum iron panel
Hyperparathyroidism	Intact PTH; serum calcium, ionized calcium, 24-hour urine for calcium
Hyperprolactinemia	Serum prolactin
Hyperthyroidism	TSH; T4 and FT1; T3
Hypogonadism	Testosterone in men; estradiol in females; LH and FSH
Hypothyroidism	TSH, T4 total, FT3, FT4, antibody tests, ferritin
Inflammatory and rheumatic diseases	Erythrocyte sedimentation rate; ANA; anti-DNA antibodies; RF
Liver disease	Liver function tests
Malabsorption	24-hour urinary calcium excretion; serum albumin level; serum calcium; serum carotene
Mastocytosis	Serum tryptase; urine N-methylhistamine; iliac bone biopsy with double tetracycline labeling

Condition	Appropriate Tests
Multiple myeloma	Serum protein electrophoresis; urine for Bence Jones proteinuria; serum calcium; intact PTH; erythrocyte sedimentation rate, alkaline phosphatase
Osteomalacia	25-hydroxyvitamin D; serum calcium
Renal disease	Serum creatinine; glomerular filtration rate
Renal tubulopathy	Urinalysis including pH; acid-base studies; urine calcium, phosphorus, amino acid, and glucose

 Different Patients, Different Tests: Alice's and Natalie's Stories

Alice is a fifty-seven-year-old postmenopausal woman with borderline osteoporosis. Because she has no history of fractures and because she eats well, exercises regularly, and does not have any digestive problems, I ordered only basic lab tests. Alice's results came back normal. Based on her health history and lab results, my recommendations included a follow-up bone density test in two years and the addition of bone-support supplements to her already healthy diet and exercise program.

Natalie is a sixty-one-year-old woman with a lumbar spine T-score of –5.0 and a hip T-score of –2.5. Over the past five years the bone density in Natalie's lumbar spine has decreased by approximately 8 percent, but nothing in her health history leaps out as an explanation for why her BMD is so dangerously low. The first test would be an X-ray of Natalie's lumbar spine along with a vertebral fracture assessment (see Chapter 3). Depending on the findings from those tests, Natalie might also need an MRI or CT scan. She should also have a comprehensive lab workup that includes all of the basic tests along with additional tests such as protein electrophoresis and tests for kidney function, parathyroid function, and bone markers. Natalie's advanced osteoporosis may be the result of one or more conditions, including bone cancer, kidney malfunction, or a primary parathyroid tumor. Some tests may need to be repeated and

additional tests required in order to get to the root of the prob-
lem. Finally, although I might order some of the preliminary
tests for Natalie, I would immediately refer her to a medical
doctor who specializes in osteoporosis and bone disease. This
patient will need medical care in addition to a bone-building
diet and exercise program.

Lab Tests: A User's Guide

Tips for Getting the Best Results

Preparation for taking a lab test can influence the results. Here a few tips to make sure your tests are as accurate as possible:

- *Fasting:* In general, it is best to take lab tests first thing in the morning after fasting for twelve hours. Research is beginning to bear this out, especially for certain assessments, including PTH and bone markers, even though fasting is not in the lab requirements for these tests. I tell my patients to always follow this procedure unless a particular test needs to be performed at different intervals during the day.

- *Exercise:* Don't exercise before getting a lab test in the morning. Walking is acceptable, but a hard workout can affect many lab tests.

- *Supplements:* In general, it is best to stop taking your supplements for twenty-four hours prior to testing. Talk with your doctor about this first as she/he may have specific reasons to keep you on supplements for certain tests or health conditions.

- *Medications:* Also check with your doctor to find out if you need to briefly stop or change the timing for taking your medications in order to get accurate lab results.

- *Read directions:* Make sure you read about the testing procedure to find out if you need to do anything in particular before testing, other than what is mentioned in these tips. It is also a good idea to ask your ordering doctor if there are any special instructions you need to know about. You can learn more about individual tests and preparation for tests at the website www.lab testsonline.com.

Testing, Testing, and Retesting

Do not hesitate to ask for lab tests to be repeated, especially if a test result seems out of line with the rest of your overall health picture. Be aware that any diagnostic testing can produce false positive or false negative results (as pointed out in Chapter 2 in regard to DXA scans). Or a lab technician could be having a bad day, causing him or her to handle specimens less carefully than required. Even with accurate results, a specimen represents only a one-day snapshot of your health. That is why sex hormone testing can be imprecise; it provides only ballpark results for hormone function. This can be true of assessments of blood calcium levels and other tests as well.

Examples of tests that I tend to order more than once when the first results come back abnormal or at the high end of normal are the PTH-intact with calcium tests, which check blood levels of parathyroid hormone and calcium. Depending on the lab, these tests can go up and down in some patients, which may be due to poor handling of the specimen. The PTH specimen should be frozen before it is sent off to be evaluated in the lab; otherwise the results are questionable. I was fortunate to be able to learn about parathyroid disease from my mentor, Claude Arnaud, MD. Many years ago, when he was monitoring a case I was handling, he had me order twelve PTH tests over a twelve-month period for a female patient. Four of her tests were in the normal range and eight were very elevated. Her blood calcium was on the high end of normal. We discovered she had a parathyroid tumor; once it was removed she gained 8 percent bone density in a two-year period. The take-away lesson from that experience was that good clinicians take into account all the information they glean from a patient's history and lab work, and will reorder tests when the diagnosis is unclear.

Finding Low-Cost Lab Tests

Although not all consumers have access to a wide variety of medical testing facilities in their locale, it nevertheless pays to shop around and compare the cost of the various procedures. In some instances there can be a big discrepancy in fees between one lab and another. Medical testing services are also available online, but like anything else found in cyberspace, it is important that the buyer beware of scams and poor-quality procedures. Of course, this holds true for any enterprise, regardless of whether it offers web-based services. In general, it's always a good idea to get referrals from reputable health practitioners or organizations and to use prudent judgment when choosing a lab-testing service.

One option for reducing lab-testing costs is to locate a licensed health-care professional who is affiliated with Professional Co-op (www.professionalco-op.com). This organization offers reasonably priced lab-testing procedures for patients of chiropractic and medical doctors, dentists, nurse practitioners, naturopaths, and acupuncture physicians. Professional Co-op is also a sponsor of Lab Tests Online (www.labtestsonline.org), a nonprofit website where patients can find a wealth of information on laboratory tests. Some alternative doctors are not permitted to order lab tests in some states. Chiropractors in California can order almost any diagnostic test, from X-rays and MRIs to laboratory tests.

Not All Labs Are Alike

Testing laboratories do not always use the same types of test kits, which means that a test conducted at one clinic can produce different results from a test conducted at another clinic, even if both assessments are done on the same day. The larger labs tend to be more standardized, but there is no guarantee of that. For example, vitamin D test results can change by as much as 25 percent from one major lab to the next. It is always a good idea to do a second test when a positive result indicates you have a problem. On occasion I send my patients to a different lab to make sure the result is accurate.

What about alternative labs that use hair analysis or other types of tests for allergies and the like? My advice is to stick with the alternative labs that have been in business for many years. Steer clear of any new test for which the lab boasts about results or makes claims that cannot be substantiated. These labs may only have a very small database, meaning they lack a broad range of "normal" results to which yours can be compared. In the Resources, you will find a list of various alternative labs that I have found to be useful.

Pursuing Good Health:
An Integrated Approach

During my years of training as a health-care practitioner, one of the guiding principles I learned is summarized in the saying "If you hear a fire alarm, don't just shut it off; look for smoke." No one would simply stop the clanging of a fire bell and ignore the fire. Rather, the fire would be extinguished, and once the immediate danger had passed the cause would be investigated. By the same token, when our bodies set off "alarms" about our bone health—whether in the form of a low bone density reading, a fracture, or a diagnosis of osteoporosis—we need to pay attention to what's causing the problem. Instead of simply squelching the symptom with medications, it is important to look at your health from as many angles as possible to create a complete, integrated picture. By moving beyond the simple measurement of a bone mineral density test and examining your health history, lab test results, and other factors that affect your health, you will be better able to understand what's *really* going in your body. Then you and your health-care provider can take steps to develop an individualized treatment program—one that includes nutrition, gastrointestinal health, and exercise as the foundation for optimizing bone health.

 KEY POINTS FROM CHAPTER 5

- It is important to rule out secondary causes of osteoporosis.
- A diagnosis of osteoporosis does not mean that bone loss is occurring presently.
- Bone loss can be the result of medications or a number of other factors.
- Sometimes it is necessary to retest lab tests.
- As a general rule, it is best to have your blood drawn for lab tests first thing in the morning after a twelve-hour fast.

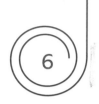

6

Osteoporosis Medications: Worth the Risks?

New prescription drugs often arrive in the marketplace surrounded by media fanfare and promotional stories about their potential benefits. In some cases the enthusiasm disappears when vast numbers of people start using them and harmful side effects become apparent. Sometimes the FDA steps in to issue cautionary guidelines, black box warnings, or outright recalls, as was the case when the diet drug Fen-Phen and the arthritis medication Vioxx were pulled off the market.

Certain drugs developed to combat osteoporosis seem to be following a similar trajectory. When first introduced in 1995, Fosamax, one of the class of drugs known as bisphosphonates, was heralded as a breakthrough in the fight against fractures. Merck, the manufacturer of Fosamax, also simultaneously worked to place thousands of DXA machines in doctor's offices for testing patients' bone density levels (see Chapter 2). Within a few years, millions of patients were taking Fosamax, even though a number of them simply had low bone density, not osteoporosis. Others were given Fosamax entirely as a preventive measure. Eventually, other bisphosphonates, such as Actonel, Boniva, and Reclast, also entered the market. To give you an idea of the size of that market, in one ten-year period Merck posted more than twenty billion dollars in worldwide sales of Fosamax.

In 2003, however, stories began to surface about a small group of cancer patients who had received bisphosphonate therapy and subsequently developed ONJ (osteonecrosis of the jaw), a condition that results in bone death in certain areas of the jaw. A few years later, the FDA alerted the public to this problem, issuing a broad, class-wide warning for all bisphosphonates. Then in 2005, reports linking bisphosphonates to atypical (low-trauma) fractures started coming to light. In a small number of patients on bisphosphonates, fractures occurred in the femur—one of the strongest bones in the body—after only minimal trauma, like being jostled on a subway train. By the spring of 2010 the mainstream media became focused on the issue, and in the fall of that year the FDA released a safety communication and required labeling changes for bisphosphonates. Patients experiencing these fractures began mounting lawsuits against Merck, the outcomes of which have been mixed or remain pending as of the publication date for this book.

As an alternative health-care practitioner who has studied bone health for decades, I viewed the initial and widespread promotion of bisphosphonates with skepticism, and I wasn't at all surprised by FDA warnings about the possible negative consequences of their use. My skepticism was based on the fact that these medications interfere with the normal process of bone turnover, which, as you may recall from Chapter 1, involves getting rid of old bone and laying down new bone. Bisphosphonates inhibit bone loss by initiating apoptosis (or regulated, "programmed" cell death) in the osteoclasts, the cells that remove old bone. Prolonged suppression of osteoclasts can result in the accumulation of old bone, and it also slows the activity of the osteoblasts that create new bone, which means less new bone is formed. Therefore, along with other health professionals, I am concerned about the potential long-term impact of bisphosphonates on bone quality.

At the same time, however, I cannot ignore the research that points to the ability of bisphosphonates to increase bone density and reduce fracture risks in some patients. After examining research such as the Fracture Intervention Trial (FIT) and other studies, I have reconsidered my opposition to bisphosphonates. When bisphosphonates are used wisely, in the appropriate situations and for a limited amount of time, they can help certain patients reduce their fracture risk.

But let me be very clear. If osteoporosis medications have been recommended to you, before making a decision about whether or not to take them, you need a full medical workup that examines your individual risk factors. As explained in Chapter 5, that workup should include a complete health history, an evaluation of your nutritional status and gastrointestinal health, and DXA tests to check your bone density in the lumbar spine, hip, and possibly the forearm. It is also essential to obtain the appropriate lab tests to help determine whether bone loss is occurring presently. And if you *are* actively losing bone, you'll want to find out if there is a reason why, so you can stop the process or slow it down.

Finally, because even the mainstream medical establishment questions the use of bisphosphonates for more than five years, the length of time you might take these particular medications—and the age at which you begin to use them—are crucial questions that must be assessed on an individual basis. Osteoporosis medications are best suited to patients who have experienced low-trauma fractures or have advanced cases of the disease.

Because all drugs have side effects and the potential for adverse reactions, the decision to use any medication involves a careful analysis of risks versus benefits for the individual patient. If you are in the process of deciding whether to use osteoporosis medications—or are already using them—this chapter will help you understand the role of bisphosphonates and other medications in a treatment plan. But whether or not you are taking medications, the disease of osteoporosis requires a multipronged approach that should *always* include paying attention to nutrition and gastrointestinal problems, and participating in exercise (if possible).

The rest of this chapter provides an overview of the medications used to treat osteoporosis. Much of the discussion focuses on the bisphosphonates, the most commonly prescribed drugs for treating osteoporosis.

How Do Osteoporosis Medications Work?

A brief review of the process of bone remodeling can give you a glimpse of how osteoporosis medications are designed to work. As explained in Chapter 1, the continuous cycle of bone remodeling involves two major bone cells: the osteoclasts, which remove old bone in a process called resorption, and the osteoblasts, which deposit new bone. (Remember: Osteo*c*lasts *c*hew up; osteo*b*lasts *b*uild up.)

Osteoporosis medications currently approved by the FDA primarily work in one of two ways. They either:

o directly or indirectly suppress the action of the osteoclasts, or

o boost the activity of the osteoblasts

The medications that suppress the osteoclasts are called "antiresorptives"—they slow the resorption process and retard bone breakdown. Bisphosphonates and a few other medications fall into this category.

The medications that promote the work of osteoblasts in building new bone are called "anabolics." To date, the only drugs in this category are teriparatide (Forteo), which is FDA-approved, and strontium ranelate (Protelos), which is not FDA approved and thus is currently unavailable for use in the United States.

Some of the most common medications used to treat osteoporosis include:

o **antiresorptives** (inhibit the removal of bone by inhibiting osteoclasts):

- *bisphosphonates*: Fosamax, Boniva, Actonel, Atelvia, Reclast, Zometa, Didronel
- *denosumab*: Prolia
- *estrogen therapy (ET)* and *hormone therapy (HT)*: various brands available
- *raloxifene* (selective estrogen receptor modulator [SERM] or estrogen agonist/antagonist): Evista
- *calcitonin**: Fortical, Miacalcin

o **anabolics** (promote the building of new bone):
- *teriparatide* (parathyroid hormone 1-34): Forteo
- *strontium ranelate*: Protelos**

---

* Though calcitonin has been prescribed to treat osteoporosis for decades, an FDA panel voted in 2013 to stop marketing it for that purpose because of cancer risks from long-term use.
** Not currently approved for use in the United States.

Basics on Bisphosphonates:
The Most Common Osteoporosis Meds

To date, bisphosphonates (BP) are the most commonly prescribed medications for treating osteoporosis. They work by interfering with the process that enables osteoclasts to remove bone, which means that less bone is broken down. During the first six to twelve months of treatment, it appears that the osteoblasts continue to form new bone, causing bone volume to increase in many patients. However, after this initial period, bone formation plateaus and slows down. For the next couple of years, the slight increases in bone density likely represent increased mineralization. However, after three to five years the BP continues to suppress osteoclasts, while the osteoblasts appear to stop active bone mineralization. Some studies have shown a dramatic decrease in bone formation after the two-year mark. This may result in the bone retaining too much old, damaged bone, resulting in poor bone quality. The atypical fractures, along with an understanding of how these medications work, gave rise to the concept of a "drug holiday," discussed later in the chapter.

Table 6.1 shows the brand and generic names for several of the most widely sold bisphosphonate medications. This class of drugs continues to proliferate, with new ones continually entering the marketplace.

Table 6.1. Common Bisphosphonate Medications for Treating Osteoporosis

Trade Name	Generic Name
Actonel; Actonel with Calcium; Atelvia	Risedronate sodium; risedronate sodium w/calcium carbonate
Boniva or Binosto	Ibandronate sodium
Fosamax; Fosamax Plus D	Alendronate sodium; alendronate sodium plus cholecalciferol (vitamin D-3)
Reclast or Zometa	Zoledronic acid

In addition to the medications listed above, other bisphosphonates are used to treat a variety of bone conditions. These include Aclasta, Aredia, Didronel, and Skelid.

Weighing the Benefits Versus the Risks

With any type of drug treatment, the fundamental question doctors and patients need to answer is whether the benefits outweigh the risks. So what are the benefits of bisphosphonates? In short, when bisphosphonates are prescribed and administered appropriately, they can stabilize or increase bone mineral density and reduce the risk of fractures. In the Fracture Intervention Trials (FIT1 and FIT2), women taking Fosamax showed a 56 percent reduction in hip fractures and a 48 percent decrease in spine fractures when evaluated by X-ray (*but see note below*). The Fracture Intervention Trial Long-Term Extension (FLEX) study followed up on participants in the original FIT research and found that the patients who remained on Fosamax (as opposed to a placebo) maintained stable bone density at the hip sites and made gains in BMD at the spine. Bisphosphonates, then, can offer benefits to patients—as long as they are given to the right patient and, as discussed below, as long as they're taken for the right length of time.

But remember that, as noted in Chapter 1, falling causes 90 percent of hip fractures. I know of some patients who chose to take bisphosphonates or other osteoporosis medications because they believed that doing so would prevent fractures, period. This is simply not the case. Although bisphosphonates can reduce fracture risk to some extent, they will not offer much protection from breaking a bone if you take a significantly hard fall. Improving balance, eliminating tripping hazards, and building bone health are crucial steps needed to substantially reduce fracture risk.

Note: The Fracture Intervention Trials mentioned above concluded that fractures were reduced by more than 50 percent for those who were taking Fosamax. How did they arrive at this number? There were thousands of women in the study group. The findings showed that 1.0 percent of those taking Fosamax experienced hip fractures when compared to the 2.2 percent of those taking placebo pills. Merck is allowed to say that the drug reduces bone fractures by 56 percent because 1.0 percent is 44 percent of 2.2 percent.

Side Effects

Because gastrointestinal problems, especially stomach cramps, are a common side effect of oral bisphosphonates, patients are advised to ingest them first thing in the morning and to remain upright and avoid eating anything for thirty to sixty minutes afterward. Oral bisphosphonates can also result in irritation of the esophagus and are not appropriate for patients with preexisting gastrointestinal problems, especially gastric reflux. Though studies linking esophageal cancer to bisphosphonate use have been conflicting, and current research is inconclusive, I have seen two patients who were diagnosed with esophageal cancer after using the oral form of these drugs for longer than five years.

Bone, joint, and muscle pain are potential side effects of all bisphosphonates, and flulike symptoms, fever, and headaches can result from receiving bisphosphonates intravenously. Bisphosphonates may also contribute to a heart rhythm disorder (atrial fibrillation) in elderly patients, but to date, no definitive link has been established. Among the rare side effects of all bisphosphonates is a condition called uveitis, which is an inflammation of the eye.

Other side effects that are thought to be rare are atypical (low-trauma) fractures of the femur and osteonecrosis of the jaw (ONJ), both of which were mentioned early in the chapter. In a study at Kaiser, a large California HMO, researchers identified 135 atypical fractures out of nearly 16,000 broken femurs. All but 3.7 percent of patients with atypical femur fractures were taking a bisphosphonate. An impending femur fracture may be signaled by deep thigh pain; some researchers estimate that in 70 percent of cases, patients reported experiencing pain or discomfort in the thigh or groin for weeks or months before fracturing their femurs. Similarly, jaw pain can be a sign of ONJ. If you are taking a bisphosphonate and are experiencing jaw pain, this should alert you to see your dentist. If you are experiencing deep thigh pain, consult with your doctor as soon as possible.

Finally, some studies suggest a problem with delayed fracture healing in patients who fracture a bone while on or after taking a bisphosphonate medication for several years. One small study reported nine patients (eight postmenopausal women and one man) who sustained unusual spontaneous nonspinal fractures while on alendronate therapy for three to eight years; six of them had delayed or absent fracture healing for three months to two years during the therapy. I've seen several patients in my own practice who have experienced delayed fracture healing while on bisphosphonates, and I strongly suspect that the medications could have been responsible for that.

I know of one doctor, Jennifer P. Schneider, MD, PhD, who experienced an atypical fracture of the femur after taking Fosamax for several years. The following is an abbreviated version of her story, in her own words. (You can hear more in an interview I conducted with her by visiting my website, www.LaniSimpson.com.)

Small Jolt, Big Fracture: Jennifer's Story

"In October 2001 I was riding on the subway in New York City when the train jolted as it pulled into a station. As I shifted my weight from my left to my right leg, I felt and heard a crack in my right thigh, and then I fell to the floor. I knew I had broken my femur. The doctors in the emergency room were mystified as to how the strongest bone in the body could just snap. I had had pain in that thigh for three months, had seen an orthopedic surgeon, and had had it X-rayed, but nothing was found. It took me several years to get an explanation. A medical article published in 2005 described several cases of unusual low-impact fractures in people on long-term Fosamax (alendronate) and suggested that the drug could have over-suppressed the normal turnover of bone, which is required to keep bones healthy... and thus [the drug] could have caused those fractures. I had been taking Fosamax for more than six years for 'osteopenia' (that is, to prevent osteoporosis). [The conclusions of that 2005 article] made sense to me. Since then, hundreds of similar cases have occurred."

As mentioned, some of the most serious adverse effects of bisphosphonate use—such as the broken femur in the case of Dr. Schneider—are thought to be rare. But they don't seem rare when they happen to you. Furthermore, I believe that the full story has not been told, simply because not enough time has passed since these drugs were introduced to allow for an adequate understanding of their effects. For example, fractures that are slow to heal or that simply do not heal are not yet listed among the side effects, yet my experience with the patients in my care leads me to believe they should be—and one day, given adequate research, they may be. The totality of the side effects of bisphosphonates is sobering. The serious adverse effects that can arise from their use underscore the need to be cautious when prescribing or accepting a prescription for them. In terms of bone health, generally speaking, bisphosphonate use is advised primarily for those who have advanced cases of osteoporosis with high fracture risk.

A Look at the Conventional Guidelines for Using Osteoporosis Drugs

Gender and age as well as individual medical conditions and fracture risk are among the factors that doctors are advised to consider when making determinations about whether to recommend medications for osteoporosis. To help doctors refine the criteria for patients who should consider these drugs, the *Clinician's Guide to Prevention and Treatment of Osteoporosis,* published by the National Osteoporosis Foundation (NOF), provides a specific set of guidelines for use with postmenopausal women and men age fifty and older.

Before prescribing medication, the NOF recommends that doctors implement the following procedures:

- o Obtain a detailed patient history pertaining to clinical risk factors for osteoporosis-related fractures and falls.

- o Perform physical examination and obtain diagnostic studies to evaluate for signs of osteoporosis and its secondary causes.

- o Modify diet/supplements and other clinical risk factors for fracture.

- o Estimate patient's ten-year probability of hip and any major osteoporosis-related fracture using the United States–adapted FRAX.

- o Make decisions on whom to treat and how to treat based on clinical judgment using this guide and all available clinical information.

Once the above steps have been completed, treatment should be *considered* for patients who meet the conditions below:

o vertebral fracture (clinical or asymptomatic) or hip fracture

o hip DXA (femoral neck or total hip) or lumbar spine T-score
  ≤ -2.5

o low bone mass (osteopenia)* and a United States–adapted
  WHO ten-year probability of a hip fracture $\geq$ 3 percent, or ten-
  year probability of any major osteoporosis-related fracture $\geq$ 20
  percent (patient preferences may indicate treatment for people
  with ten-year fracture probabilities above or below these levels)

Adherence to the NOF guidelines—especially the recommendation to take a detailed patient history—enables both doctors and patients to make informed decisions about treatment. In my experience, I have found that most health practitioners do not follow these
steps. For example, as discussed in previous chapters, some doctors
prescribe osteoporosis medications based on the results of one DXA
test, without getting a full history or considering possible underlying
conditions. And some doctors don't fully appreciate or understand
the impact of nutrition and exercise on bone health. In addition, an
initial bone-health assessment should take between sixty and ninety
minutes, yet in a managed-care system most doctors spend no more
than fifteen minutes with each patient. If you find yourself in this
situation, consider getting a second opinion from a practitioner who
specializes in bone health and who is willing to take the time needed
to evaluate your individual case. Please also know that you may need
to work with more than one professional in order to have your case
evaluated appropriately.

Are the Conventional Guidelines Sufficient?

Although the NOF guidelines are useful, any number of other factors
can affect whether an individual patient should consider osteoporosis
medications. For example, according to the conventional guidelines

* This NOF guideline refers to "bone mass," which, in this context, has the same
meaning as the term "bone density" used throughout this book. As also discussed
throughout the book, the term "osteopenia" does not refer to a disease condition,
and the current, preferred description is simply "low bone density."

described above, a seventy-year-old woman with a T-score of –2.5 would seem a likely candidate for osteoporosis medications. But if she has never fractured and has no other risk factors, such an intervention may be unnecessary—and if it is unnecessary it may do more harm than good.

In other cases, the decision to begin medications is relatively clear-cut. Suppose a patient is seventy years old, has a T-score in the –4.0 range or lower, and has also experienced two low-trauma fractures. In this case, osteoporosis medications should definitely be considered. However, when a patient falls into the borderline area—for example, if he or she has a T-score of –2.5 but no other significant risk factors and is under age sixty—then pharmacologic treatment is *highly* questionable.

Generally speaking, some of the main factors to consider when evaluating the appropriateness of osteoporosis medications include:

○ *Presence or absence of active bone loss:* This is a crucial factor that must be evaluated before starting any treatment regimen. Are you losing bone now? If not, your bone is stable, and, depending on your current bone density levels and risk factors, you may have no need for medications. T-score measurements play an important role in doctors' decisions related to osteoporosis medications. But no matter what the T-scores show—even if they indicate a diagnosis of osteoporosis—a *single* DXA test cannot determine whether a patient is actively losing bone.

○ *Lab test results:* The NOF recommends that osteoporosis medications not be prescribed until secondary causes of bone loss are ruled out through appropriate lab testing. This recommendation is particularly important. Besides identifying or eliminating possible underlying causes of osteoporosis, lab work is also needed to help determine whether active bone loss is occurring. These tests will often include bone markers and a twenty-four-hour urine collection.

○ *FRAX limitations:* The NOF suggests that FRAX results be considered before doctors prescribe medications. But remember, FRAX has significant limitations (as described in Chapter 4), so this tool should be viewed as giving us only one piece of a patient's overall bone-health picture.

o *Cause of prior fractures:* The NOF recommends that osteoporosis medications be considered for those with a current or prior vertebral or hip fracture. Although the presence of fractures may be a main factor in decisions related to pharmacological interventions, fracturing because of a severe accident is different from sustaining a low-trauma osteoporosis fracture. The cause of any fracture needs to be weighed carefully in assessing one's present bone health and the possible use of medications.

o *Will medication reduce the risk for fractures? And if so, to what extent?* Any decision to take osteoporosis medications should be informed by a practical understanding of the benefits you might receive from the drugs. You also need to understand how long the benefits might last. Most importantly, when you stop taking certain osteoporosis medications, bone loss often recurs within the first one to three years. The fact that you can lose the bone you gained should help you see the importance of making sure there is no secondary cause for your bone loss—and if there is, of determining whether it is being properly managed.

Remember, the whole point of using osteoporosis medications is to reduce your risk for fractures—so be sure to have a clear picture of your fracture risk before you include these drugs as part of your treatment regimen. Also make sure you understand how much fracture reduction you can expect from a medication or treatment program of any kind.

As discussed, balance, body size, and height can all have an impact on fracture risk. If you have good balance and you're mindful of your body and its relationship to the surrounding environment, your risk for fracturing is lower than it is for someone with poor balance and limited body awareness. Taller people may have a higher fracture risk simply because any fall they take will have more impact than a fall by a shorter person. And, as described in the list of risk factors provided in Chapter 4, those with a low body weight or smaller bones are at greater risk for fractures.

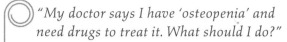

"My doctor says I have 'osteopenia' and need drugs to treat it. What should I do?"

As pointed out in Chapter 3, "osteopenia" refers simply to low bone density as reflected by T-scores between –1.0 and –2.4. T-scores in this range do not necessarily indicate disease, and the term "osteopenia" was never meant to serve as a diagnosis. At the time the word gained currency, in the mid-1990s, widespread advertising for Fosamax and other bisphosphonates convinced many women and their doctors that these drugs were appropriate for preventing future fractures, even in patients who were healthy and had no or few risk factors for osteoporosis. That practice is diminishing, but there are still physicians who prescribe medications solely on the basis of low bone density scores.

Again, before a treatment plan is developed, the crucial factor to consider is whether or not active bone loss is taking place. This can be assessed by comparing two accurately acquired DXA tests and through lab testing. Suppose, for example, that at age forty-eight your bone density measured at –1.3, and at age fifty-two it measured at –2.4. Both of these T-scores are in the low bone density range, and the follow-up reading indicates that a significant amount of bone has been lost (about 12 percent), so there is cause for concern. Still, rather than automatically treating the condition with osteoporosis medications, further evaluation is needed to determine whether there is a secondary cause for the bone loss, such as hyperparathyroidism, lack of exercise, or deficiency of a nutrient such as calcium or vitamin D. Alternatively, bone loss in women may result from hormone depletion at menopause or the onset of menopause, for which treatment using bioidentical hormones can be considered. Regardless of the cause of a person's bone loss, or even if the cause is identifiable, it may be minimized or stopped altogether using more natural means rather than osteoporosis medications.

The bottom line: If your doctor has prescribed an osteoporosis medication based solely on low bone density scores, use the information found in the preceding chapters to guide you in obtaining

> a more complete workup of your case, including additional diag-
> nostic testing if applicable. Also be sure to take action to support
> your bone health, as recommended in the book's later chapters.

The Bisphosphonate Debate: How Long Can a Person Safely Use Them?

In 2012 the *New England Journal of Medicine* published an FDA review of the clinical studies measuring the effectiveness of long-term bisphosphonate use. According to an FDA Consumer Update, "[S]ome patients may be able to stop using bisphosphonates after three to five years and still continue to benefit from their use." Marcea Whitaker, MD, from the FDA's Center for Drug Evaluation and Research, summarized the findings from the review by saying, "These drugs clearly work. We just don't know yet the optimum period of time individual patients should be on the drug to both maximize its effectiveness and minimize potential risks."

Even before the FDA released its review, Susan Ott, MD, a professor of medicine at the University of Washington, clearly stated the case for putting time limits on the use of bisphosphonates in a paper for the *Cleveland Clinic Journal of Medicine*. Dr. Ott's paper pointed out some of the risks associated with long-term bisphosphonate use and highlighted the following results from studies of the drugs, findings that other researchers have also noted:

o There is accumulating evidence that the risk of atypical fracture of the femur increases after five years of bisphosphonate use.

o Most of the data on the safety and efficacy of bisphosphonate treatment for osteoporosis are from patients who took the drug for less than five years.

o Research shows that bisphosphonates are retained to some extent in the skeleton throughout the course of the patient's life.

o The use of bisphosphonates to treat women with low bone density (or osteopenia) is "based on hope, not evidence."

Given the risks associated with bisphosphonate use, along with the fact that they are retained in the bones long after patients stop taking them, setting limits as to the length of time they are used is appropriate. As Dr. Ott put it, "[I]t is reasonable to stop bisphosphonates after five years of use and then to follow patients with markers of bone turnover. As long as the levels of these markers remain reduced, adding an antiresorptive drug does not make physiologic sense."

Researchers, government agencies, and pharmaceutical companies will continue to hash out the issues surrounding the safety and effectiveness of long-term bisphosphonate use. Meanwhile, where does this leave the average patient? Most likely, the five-year time frame on the use of these medications will become more common. If that is the case—assuming that bisphosphonates are appropriate for you in the first place—when should you begin taking them? For example, suppose you take a bisphosphonate for five years during your mid-fifties in the hope of preventing fractures when you are older. What will you do when you actually *are* older? You have already used the drug for the maximum length of time suggested by researchers and other experts. Will starting an additional course be effective—and safe—should you and your doctor decide that you need it later in life? No one knows the precise answer to this question because not enough time has passed for adequate research on the effects of using these drugs in an on-again, off-again regimen over the course of many years or even decades.

We do know that bisphosphonates suppress the activity of the cells that break down old bone, and there is mounting evidence that bisphosphonates can impact bone quality over the long term, putting some people at increased risk for fractures. It therefore seems that the safest and most reasonable approach would be to avoid using them until and unless they are necessary—and the later you start to use them, the better. Generally speaking, bisphosphonates can be considered for those who are both at a moderate to high risk for fracturing and unable to use other treatment modalities because they have been exhausted or would likely be ineffective.

As with any question about how long to use a medication—or whether to use it at all—patients are best advised to choose a healthcare provider who will closely evaluate all of the information about their bone health. Only then are they in a position to make informed decisions about when or if bisphosphonates are appropriate for them.

I have seen the benefits of BPs when they are prescribed to the right patients.

What About Taking a "Drug Holiday"?

The concept of having osteoporosis patients take a "holiday" from bisphosphonates began to emerge around the time researchers started making the connection between the use of the drugs and the development of osteonecrosis of the jaw and atypical fractures of the femur.

Working from the premise that bisphosphonates remain active in the bone for approximately two years after a patient stops taking them—unlike other types of osteoporosis drugs—researchers started to investigate the amount of time the active effects (i.e., suppression of osteoclasts) continue once the medication is stopped. As yet, studies have not established who should or should not be considered for a drug holiday. For instance:* One study at Loyola University showed that bone density remained stable for three years in patients who stopped taking bisphosphonates. Study investigator Dr. Pauline Camacho told Reuters in 2011, "We are stopping the drugs, but we don't know how long patients should be off them."

It's important to keep in mind that the idea of a drug holiday gained attention as a potential solution to the problem of the more serious side effects mentioned earlier, including osteonecrosis of the jaw and atypical fractures of the femur. But I question whether it is an appropriate solution. Conventional medicine recognizes the importance of setting time limits on bisphosphonate use. In my opinion, however, much of the thinking about the issue does not go far enough. Serious side effects have been reported after five years of bisphosphonate use; therefore, I think it is wise to consider a drug holiday after two to three years.

It is crucial for health-care providers to conduct proper lab tests, including tests for bone markers, before and during treatment. If a

* Another study of long-term bisphosphonate use, published in the *Journal of Clinical Endocrinology* and led by Nelson B. Watts, recommended a break in treatment after patients had taken the drugs for five to ten years, depending on the individual's level of fracture risk. Watts wrote, "Although there is no strong science to guide us, we believe that some time off treatment should be offered to most patients on long-term bisphosphonate therapy."

break in treatment is implemented, it should continue until and un-less bone loss begins to recur based on lab findings. Further, some practitioners advise a drug holiday rather than addressing secondary causes of bone loss, such as an abysmal diet or a digestive issue. In fact, resolving these secondary issues could result in stabilizing and im-proving the patient's bone health far better than taking time off from a bisphosphonate regimen. In addition, as we have learned, a significant number of patients who take the medications—such as those who were diagnosed with "osteopenia" with no additional risk factors or questionable risk factors—never needed them in the first place. For these patients, stopping the drug permanently is likely called for.

No evidence currently exists showing that the risks associated with long-term use of bisphosphonates can be mitigated via a drug holiday. Will taking time away from the drugs—only to use them again at a later date—resolve the problem of adverse side effects? At this point, no one knows. To date, there has been no research on the impact of intermittent bisphosphonate use over many years. Although at this point the drug holiday is a reasonable response to the risks associated with BP use, any assumption that temporarily stopping the drug regi-men can mitigate its effect on bone quality over years of on-again, off-again use is purely guesswork.

Finally, the fact that bisphosphonates should not be taken indefi-nitely underscores the point that they should not be prescribed in-discriminately. Again, osteoporosis medications should primarily be considered in advanced cases of the disease, especially when fracture risk is high.

What about switching from a bisphosphonate to another osteopo-rosis medication as a sort of drug holiday to avoid the risks associated with bisphosphonate use? I often see patients whose medical doctors switched their medications because the patients expressed concerns about the drugs they were taking. All too often the "new" medication is not new at all because it is in the same category as the original. A good example is a switch from Fosamax to Boniva, both of which are bisphosphonates. Or maybe after a patient has spent five years on Fosamax, her or his doctor prescribes Prolia. Although it is not a bisphosphonate, Prolia is still an antiresorptive; that is, it ultimately ends up suppressing osteoclasts, which means the new prescription is not a true switch. Remember, a holiday from osteoporosis medications is intended to reduce the risk of adverse effects by providing a break in the drugs' oversuppression of osteoclasts (the cells that remove bone tissue).

If your doctor agrees to, or suggests, changing your medication, be sure to find out exactly what category the new drug falls into. Is it a bisphosphonate or one of the other antiresorptives? Or is it an anabolic medication? Be sure to understand the pros and cons of any new medication before agreeing to change.

The choice to start or stop taking any medication should not be made lightly or without a thorough evaluation of your health needs. Such an evaluation should include your discussing the issue with an informed, trusted health care professional who knows your medical history. Furthermore, abruptly ceasing a prescribed medication—as opposed to reducing the dosage gradually—can have serious medical consequences. It is especially important to consult your provider when you are considering going off osteoporosis medications. Bisphosphonates, as noted, remain active in the bone for a period of time after you stop taking them, but other types of osteoporosis medications do not. This means that within a year of stopping some medications you may lose the bone you gained (assuming you gained any). Bone loss following bisphosphonate use can resume after approximately two years.

Don't make decisions about drugs based on one article you may have read online or on a neighbor's story about a good or bad experience with a medication. Your body and your health needs are *unique to you*. Seek out the answers that will help you make informed decisions about the care *you* require.

The Non-Bisphosphonates: Other Osteoporosis Medications

In addition to bisphosphonates, several other medications are included in the category of antiresorptives—that is, they work by preventing osteoclasts from getting rid of old bone. This section offers an overview of these medications as well as a discussion of teriparatide

(Forteo), the one FDA-approved medication that boosts the osteo-blasts' ability to build new bone.

Note: Keep in mind non-bisphosphonate drugs do not linger in the bones as bisphosphonates do. This means that bone loss can occur more quickly after discontinuing these medications.

Teriparatide (Forteo)

Teriparatide (brand name Forteo) is a synthetic parathyroid hormone. It is the one FDA-approved drug among those listed for treatment of osteoporosis that is classified as an anabolic medication—meaning it promotes the bone-building work of the osteoblasts. Interestingly, this drug stimulates both osteoclasts and osteoblasts. The osteoblasts outpace the osteoclasts, however, and the net result is fresh new bone.

Forteo is typically reserved for patients with advanced cases of osteoporosis who have a high fracture risk, especially those who have sustained osteoporosis-related fractures. The general duration of treatment is eighteen months to two years and requires a daily in-jection. Some studies show fracture reductions of 65 percent in those who took Forteo for the recommended amount of time. In order to maintain the new bone, it is recommended that patients take a bis-phosphonate or Prolia for two years following Forteo treatment. If patients do not take either follow-up medication, the bone gained by using Forteo *will be lost,* often within a two-year period. Presently, Forteo can only be used for a maximum of two years. At some point it will likely be available for longer periods of treatment or for sporadic use over subsequent years.

Forteo is one of the only options for people who have been on bisphosphonates for an extended period of time (typically over five years) and who are experiencing nontraumatic fractures or have frac-tures that are not healing well. It is horrible that some people are in this situation. I have had several patients who were saved from the ravages of being on bisphosphonates for too long by switching to Forteo. The drug literally turned their situation around, healing their fractures and improving their overall bone density and bone health.

Leg cramps and dizziness are two of Forteo's many side effects. The drug may also contribute to modest elevations in serum and urine calcium, though there appears to be no risk of kidney stones developing as a result. In animal studies, Forteo showed an increase in osteosarcoma, a type of bone cancer that is typically expressed in adolescence and is therefore not a likely risk for adults. Forteo is not recommended for people who have bone cancer or who are at risk for bone metastasis. If you have had cancer, visit the Forteo website for an update regarding this issue. Some doctors are recommending Forteo for advanced cases of osteoporosis in patients who are five to ten years postcancer.

Back in the late 1990s I was privileged to be mentored by Claude Arnaud, MD, one of the researchers who developed Forteo. I was privy to the early results of the drug's testing and witnessed the excitement about its potential. More than two million people have taken Forteo over the past ten years, and the drug has proved exceptionally effective. It provided a significant benefit for Dr. Jennifer Schneider, whose story appears earlier in this chapter. Her atypical fracture, which remained unhealed long after healing should have occurred, was finally able to mend once she included Forteo as part of her treatment regimen.

Denosumab (Prolia)

Denosumab, marketed under the brand name Prolia, is categorized as an antiresorptive medication. Like the bisphosphonates, Prolia prevents osteoclasts from removing old and damaged bone. Instead of suppressing already mature osteoclasts (which is what the bisphosphonates do), it prevents the precursor cells for osteoclasts from developing into mature osteoclasts. Prolia does this by latching on to the cellular "messengers" from osteoblasts that "tell" the osteoclasts to start removing old bone. By scrambling the messages, the drug prevents the formation of osteoclasts, which interferes with their function and survival. Because of its ability to inhibit cellular activities, Prolia is categorized as a RANK ligand (RANKL) inhibitor (and is also technically labeled a human monoclonal antibody).

The FDA approved this drug in 2010 for use in postmenopausal women and in men who are at high risk of fracture, as well as for those receiving certain cancer treatments. Patients taking Prolia visit the doctor's office every six months for an injection. They must have a blood test prior to each dose to make certain their blood calcium levels are normal. If calcium levels are low, they must be corrected before the patient can receive the injection of Prolia.

Some of the more troubling side effects of Prolia are the same as those for bisphosphonates. Cases of atypical femur fractures and ONJ have been reported. Remember, this drug is relatively new and in an entirely new class. Researchers won't know all of its side effects until thousands of people have used it for years.

One of my main concerns regarding Prolia is its impact on the immune system. It suppresses the immune system by binding with T-cells and B-cells, and serious infections are more common in people who take Prolia as opposed to a placebo. This seems to occur in a very small percentage of people; however, anyone with lowered immune function needs to carefully weigh the drug's potential benefits and risks.

Results from clinical trials showed that Prolia reduced the incidence of new spine fractures by 68 percent and hip fractures by 40 percent over three years. This does not mean, however, that in ten years patients will continue to experience the same reduction in fracture rates. Patients should also note that Prolia does not remain in the bones, and once they stop taking it they will likely lose what they have gained unless other measures are in place to maintain bone density.

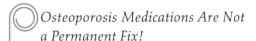

Osteoporosis Medications Are Not a Permanent Fix!

The problem with osteoporosis medications is that patients can lose the bone they gained within one to three years after discontinuing the drug. This is one reason why nutrition, gastrointestinal health, and exercise should form a strong foundation for a more holistic approach in the treatment of osteoporosis.

Hormone Therapy

The loss of estrogen at menopause clearly leads to bone loss for most women in the subsequent years. For decades, doctors prescribed estrogen to women to counteract this loss. "ET," or "estrogen therapy," refs to the use of estrogen alone. "HT" stands for "hormone therapy," which typically includes estrogen combined with progesterone and, in some instances, testosterone. You may also have heard the term "bioidentical hormones," which means hormones that are identical to the ones the human body produces. This is a preferred treatment option you will learn more about in Chapter 8.

Both ET and HT have been shown to increase bone density in the spine and hip and reduce the risk of spine and hip fractures. In 2002, however, the massive national research study known as the Women's Health Initiative (WHI) found that the increased risks of breast cancer, heart attack, blood clots, and mental decline outweighed the benefits of reduced fractures among women taking Prempro, a combination of Premarin, which consists of estrogens derived from horse urine, and Provera, a nonbioidentical form of progesterone. Another wing of the study using estrogen only (Premarin) *did not* find the same risk as the hormonal combo contained in Prempro. As it turns out, the nonbioidentical progesterone was responsible for most of the side effects. Estrogen in the form of estradiol can help *prevent* postmenopausal bone loss, but it is not considered a treatment for osteoporosis.

Tablets, transdermal skin patches, and other forms of HT are available in a wide variety of dosage levels from numerous manufacturers, and side effects may vary. Patients need to discuss the use of these medications with their health-care provider.

Although the relationship between male hormones and fracture risk is not entirely clear, hormone therapy may be appropriate for certain men because low testosterone levels can affect bone health. Men with osteoporosis may be candidates for testosterone replacement therapy if blood tests or other symptoms indicate that the treatment might be beneficial.

My opinion: Hormone therapy is a reasonable choice for women who have low bone density or osteoporosis, especially during the years surrounding menopause, and who have no contraindications such as estrogen-related breast cancer in their health history. The use of HT has been shown to aid in the stabilization of bone loss prior to and during menopause.

Raloxifene (Evista)

Researchers looking for a compound that would tap the beneficial effects of estrogen therapy while minimizing its potential risks developed raloxifene (brand name Evista), which is an estrogen agonist/ antagonist. In the past, it was also labeled as a selective estrogen receptor modulator, or SERM.

Neither a hormone nor an estrogen, raloxifene acts like estrogen in some tissues, but it works as an estrogen antagonist in others. In terms of osteoporosis treatment, raloxifene is an antiresorptive. It has been shown to minimally reduce the risk of spine fractures, but there are no data on its ability to reduce hip fractures. Raloxifene was originally developed as an anti–breast cancer medication; studies have shown that it can decrease the risk of breast cancer by a small percentage.

The pill form of Evista is taken once a day. Some possible side effects include hot flashes, leg cramps, deep vein thrombosis, and, in a small percentage of women, an increase in rates of endometrial cancer. Some doctors recommend this drug for women who have been diagnosed with estrogen-positive breast cancer, especially when bone loss is a concern.

Calcitonin (Miacalcin, Fortical)

Calcitonin is a natural hormone produced in the thyroid gland. One of its functions is to retard the activity of osteoclasts, meaning it decreases the breakdown of bone. Calcitonin products include Miacalcin, which is sold in injectable form and as a nasal spray, and Fortical, a nasal spray.

Calcitonin is used to treat symptomatic Paget's disease of the bone (which causes oversized, misshapen bones) and hypercalcemia (an excess of calcium in the blood). In the past, calcitonin had FDA approval for use in treating osteoporosis, but in March of 2013 an FDA advisory panel voted that the agency no longer support the marketing of calcitonin as a treatment for osteoporosis because the risks outweighed the benefits. Two studies concluded that those who took calcitonin showed higher rates of cancer than those who did not take the drug. The panel also advised that future studies investigate whether or not the drug can reduce fracture risk; if so, it may still have a limited use for osteoporosis patients who are unable to take other medications.

Non–FDA Approved Medications

Some medications have been approved in other countries for the treatment of osteoporosis but haven't received FDA approval for that use in the United States. Here's a quick look at a few of them:

- *Strontium ranelate (SR):* Approved for osteoporosis treatment in Europe and Canada, SR is classified as an anabolic medication because it stimulates osteoblasts to build new bone. It appears to simultaneously increase bone formation and decrease bone resorption, thus resulting in the creation of new bone. Specifically, the dual mode of action of SR is due to direct effects on both osteoblasts and osteoclasts, as reflected by the changes in bone markers in clinical trials. In early 2013, warnings about SR's association with heart problems began to emerge. In addition, this medication is taken up by the bone (replacing calcium) and remains there to some extent throughout one's life, and we don't know what impact this may have on bone quality over time. Doctors in Europe are now more cautious about prescribing this medication.

- *Etidronate, pamidronate, tiludronate:* These bisphosphonates may be used to treat other conditions such as Paget's disease, which can cause areas of osteoporosis.

- *Sodium fluoride (SF):* SF can apparently stimulate new bone formation, though the evidence is conflicting and highly controversial. In addition, SF replaces calcium in bone. Many years ago, women who were treated with high doses of fluoride did experience an increase in bone density, but they also experienced more fractures much later, indicating that the bone quality was poor.

The following medications have been approved in Europe for treatment of osteoporosis, but not yet in the United States:

- *Parathyroid hormone 1-84 (PTH 1-84):* Shown in one clinical study to reduce the risk of vertebral fractures, this form of PTH may be available in the United States in the future. A study published in the *Journal of Bone and Mineral Research* (April 2013) concluded that PTH 1-84 may reduce the strength of peripheral bones, whereas Forteo (PTH 1-34) preserves that strength.

o *Tibolone:* A synthetic steroid hormone, tibolone is currently prescribed for patients in Europe for the treatment of osteoporosis. The studies supporting it as an osteoporosis therapy are scant, and its use is not recommended.

Weighing the Risks

Given the huge potential market for osteoporosis medications, researchers and pharmaceutical companies are actively engaged in developing new approaches to treatment. Keep in mind that many more osteoporosis medications will come down the pike. One of the most exciting areas of research today is looking at more ways to increase anabolic activity; that is, stimulating the osteoblasts to lay down new healthy bone. However, the fact that a medication is new is cause for concern. Sometimes it takes years after a drug has been released to see risk factors that were not understood in the initial studies. As mentioned at the start of this chapter, some drugs are recalled years after their initial release due to severe side effects.

At the risk of sounding like a broken record, I have emphasized that the core elements of any osteoporosis treatment plan should incorporate proper nutrition (including vitamin and mineral supplements) and exercise. But despite the benefits of nutrition and exercise, which are essential to building healthy bone and stabilizing bone loss, in my opinion, some patients will need to consider taking osteoporosis medications. That's especially true for patients with advanced cases of the disease. If you are in this situation, be sure that you understand and weigh the risks and benefits associated with these drugs. When used properly, they may provide the boost your bones need to prevent fractures. Any choice to take them, however, should be made after carefully weighing the potential risks and benefits in your particular case.

For individuals for whom osteoporosis drugs are truly indicated, combining them with nutrition and exercise can provide real benefits.

Dr. Keith McCormick, an alternative health practitioner and athlete, was diagnosed with osteoporosis in his forties. He is a good example of someone who benefitted from a balance of conventional medications and more natural interventions.

Osteoporosis Medications Can Make a Difference: Keith's Story

Keith McCormick is a chiropractic physician, a pentathlete, and an ex-Olympian. Having pursued a healthy lifestyle for most of his life, he seemed one of the least likely people to be diagnosed with osteoporosis in his mid-forties. Yet he was. The diagnosis, and the multiple fractures he experienced within a five-year period, caused him to investigate why he had the disease and what he could do to stop the fractures.

Though he describes his doctors as caring and patient, Mc-Cormick also found they could offer him little more than prescriptions for Fosamax and calcium. So he set out to develop a nutritional program to help strengthen his bones. Because his case was severe enough that lifestyle enhancements alone would not have allowed his bone to stabilize as quickly as was needed, he also took Forteo and Fosamax for a period of time to stop his fractures and stabilize his bone. In his case, his recovery was enhanced because he was open to the benefits of osteoporosis drugs. He coupled his use of medications with a commitment to doing everything he could to strengthen his bones through natural methods, a combination that enabled him to improve both his bone density and his bone quality. McCormick shares his nutritional approach and other lessons he learned about bone health in his book, The Whole-Body Approach to Osteoporosis.

KEY POINTS FROM CHAPTER 6

- Medications are often prescribed when patients do not need them.
- Osteoporosis medications can result in serious side effects.

o When medications are given to patients who need them, they can be beneficial.

o There is no free lunch. Medications can have serious side effects, but for some patients, the risk of not taking medications may be greater than the risk of taking them.

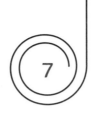

Alternatives to Medications: An Integrative Approach to Bone Health

As we saw in Chapter 6, osteoporosis medications are not the panacea that some people believe them to be. Given some of the drugs' serious side effects, I have a great deal of empathy for consumers who are attracted to alternatives to the remedies offered by conventional medicine. In my opinion, the best approach to treating or preventing osteoporosis does not rely solely on either conventional or "alternative" medicine, but instead integrates the two as appropriate.

What Do We Mean by "Integrative Medicine"?

An approach to health care that has been popularized by Andrew Weil and Deepak Chopra, integrative medicine focuses on treating the person as a whole. It considers lifestyle, mind, and body as integral components to a complete view of health. This approach makes a lot of sense when we consider how our bodies function. For example, the digestive organs break down food and absorb nutrients so that the entire body can be nourished. (As you'll see in Chapter 9, digestive dysfunction can lead to serious problems elsewhere in the body, including in the bones.) As another example, endocrine glands in various parts of the body produce hormones—also known as chemical "messengers"—that affect cells in other parts of the body. (And as you'll see in Chapter 8, the hormones direct many key aspects of the body's functioning; for example, reproduction, metabolism, and bone growth.) Of course, it is not just the physical body that works as a unit. Research shows that our thoughts and feelings have an impact on our physical health; changes in our thinking can lead to changes in both our emotions and our behavior. We are complex beings, and each aspect of ourselves is affected by every other aspect. Integrative medicine takes this complexity into account, viewing the body as a unified system rather than a collection of separate parts.

Consistent with a holistic approach, integrative medicine blends the best of the conventional and "alternative" worlds. (Some people prefer the term "complementary" to "alternative." Strictly speaking, "complementary treatment" refers to a treatment used *in conjunction with* conventional medicine, while "alternative treatment" refers to one used *in place of* conventional medicine, but many people use the terms interchangeably.) Stated in a slightly different way, integrative medicine involves treating health conditions using both natural means and the resources of Western medicine when necessary. Integrative medicine, then, is more than alternative medicine. The integrative approach is offered by a range of practitioners, including naturopaths, chiropractors, acupuncturists, some medical doctors, and others. And here's some really good news: Studies show that bone health depends on many of the factors that practitioners of integrative medicine focus on, for example, diet, gastrointestinal health, regular exercise, "nerve flow" (the uninterrupted "flow" of nerve activity), and stress reduction—all of which are discussed in more detail in later chapters.

Bone health needs to be assessed from a comprehensive or holistic point of view. The conventional medical recommendation for dealing with osteoporosis—"Take this pill, drink milk, and take Tums"—is *woefully* inadequate! But if you decide to venture into the world of alternative bone-health treatments, the information found there can be inadequate as well. You may read, for example, about diets or nutritional supplements that claim to improve bone density or reverse osteoporosis. Even if a particular supplement does, in fact, help increase bone health for some people, how do you know that it is a supplement *you* need? Or if a good friend tells you that she has decided to become a vegan because vegans have better bones, should you consider the diet for yourself? Do vegans in fact have stronger bones? Another friend may tell you that a book he read claims that if he does yoga daily, he will gain 1 percent bone mass each year for the next ten years. Is this claim accurate? How can you tell the legitimate bone-building remedies from approaches that play on wishful thinking?

It's important to distinguish between valid and bogus claims, yet the alternative health practices and products that can help you maintain and strengthen your bones are not always subject to double-blind clinical trials or other rigorous assessments. *Perhaps most important, whether the treatment you're considering is alternative or conventional, there is no "magic bullet" cure for osteoporosis.* There are no quick fixes when it comes to treating this disease. You learned in Chapter 5 that each patient should be looked at individually due to the wide range of factors that contribute to osteoporosis. The circumstances that cause the condition in one person are not necessarily the same as those that cause it in someone else. And just as there is no one factor that *causes* osteoporosis, there is no one treatment for it.

What should you do if you want to incorporate alternative bone-building treatments into your bone-health plan? This chapter gives you the information you need to research alternatives well and wisely, with both skepticism and openness. Not every recommendation you come across will be right for you, but you may find some that are. A few of the more common alternative treatments for osteoporosis are discussed later in the chapter. First, though, I want to share some information that will help you to steer clear of false claims.

There Are Alternative Therapies, but There Are No Miracles

Perhaps you have seen ads on the Internet or elsewhere claiming that a certain alternative treatment will give you unprecedented increases in bone density or even reverse your osteoporosis altogether. There may be studies that appear to support the claim—a team of scientists, say, proudly displaying the product or treatment, and beautiful graphs that "show" the effect of the intervention. Be very wary of "miracle" cures, because they are not legitimate. Testimonials can be false, too.

It is not unheard of for a company to post a testimonial that is untrue; in fact, some companies "buy" testimonials from writers who are hired specifically for that purpose. Sadly, there is no miracle cure for osteoporosis, and any claim suggesting that there is stretches the truth significantly.

I share some of my personal experiences with "miracle cures" later in this chapter, but for now, know that bone-building is a slow, complex process. Increases in bone density aren't gained quickly or easily. Claiming that rapid and significant gains can occur based on the use of one or two interventions is like claiming that a four-thousand-square-foot home can be built in a day, with only a shovel and cement. Still, with changes in diet or the replenishing of deficient nutrients, the bones can begin to strengthen, and bone density may increase as well.

Stand-Alone Alternative Treatments: Can They Reverse Osteoporosis?

Some of the alternative osteoporosis treatments you will most likely encounter include strontium citrate, lactoferrin, natural progesterone, numerous expensive calcium products, and various exercise routines. It is true that some of these alternatives may increase bone strength and bone density. And this means, in turn, that there may be some truth to the claims advertisers make. On the other hand, as I write this book *I am unaware of any product or activity that will significantly increase bone density on its own.*

Be wary of companies, testimonials, or even trusted friends who report major success based solely on the use of a specific product. Some advertisers claim that their product results in bone density gains of more than 10 percent over the course of only one year. I have yet to see such a fantastic gain. Various websites post testimonials from consumers and patients who claim that their osteoporosis has completely reversed. I have contacted many of these companies and many of the individuals whose results they promote in an attempt to verify the claims, and never has anyone been able to provide me with solid, statistically valid proof that their bone density changed for the better based on the product in question. Below, I share some of my personal experience with these false—or at best, overstated—success stories.

Exaggerated success with a lactoferrin-based product: A doctor contacted me to share his belief that lactoferrin (a protein found in milk) would significantly increase bone density or even reverse osteoporosis. The company that he bought his products from seemed credible, so I talked with one of the doctors who represented the supplement. He told me that his eighty-five-year-old aunt had gained a whopping 25 percent bone mass in her spine after one year of taking the product. He sent me her bone density tests as "proof," but the test results were unreliable and inaccurate. For one thing, the second test was taken *two* years after the first test, not one—but more important, the testing was conducted at two different facilities and on two different types of machines. As you learned in Chapter 2, comparisons of bone density tests are unreliable unless the tests are conducted on the same machine. Finally, even if the patient did experience a gain in bone density, the increase was more likely due to her physical condition, not the supplement she was taking. She had severe osteoarthritis in her spine, a condition that can make it appear that bone density has increased when in fact it has not.

Questionable effectiveness of a Chinese herbal supplement: Not long ago, an acupuncturist contacted me to tell me about a product consisting of a proprietary blend of Chinese herbs. His father had developed the original formula, which was designed to *pull calcium from the arteries and put it back into the bone*—yikes! He said that while no studies had been done, he had five patients for whom the product had resulted in increases in bone density, and he had the scans to prove it. His proof, though, was highly problematic. He had compared the right hip to the left in one case; in another, the bone density tests were conducted using two different machines; and the results in the third case were within the 2 percent margin of error for bone density testing. (Remember, even if your second test is on the same type of machine—or on the exact same machine—as your first test, you have to see a 3 to 5 percent change in bone density before you can accept it as real.) Finally, the acupuncturist's remaining two cases were simply not diagnostic, as his patients had been improperly positioned on the scanning table. Essentially, the acupuncturist had no proof whatsoever that his product did what he thought it did.

False osteoporosis "reversal": About five years ago I ran across a blog whose author claimed to have significantly increased her bone density as the result of a particular diet and exercise program. I was very interested in the report, so I contacted her and she agreed to send me the results of her DXA tests as proof of the success of her program. After reviewing her case, I found that she had *not* reversed her osteoporosis; instead, she had a very advanced case. In addition, one of her lumbar vertebrae showed a 50 percent reduction in height, an indication that the bone had fractured. The woman was unaware that she had sustained a fracture, and there was no mention of it in the DXA report. When I asked her whether she had had any low back pain within the past three years, she reported that a year earlier she had suffered a significant bout of low back pain that subsided after six weeks—about the length of time it takes for a fracture to heal. As with osteoarthritis, fractures can result in false increases in bone density. This woman's higher test scores were due primarily to her fracture.

Buying into misleading progesterone claims: In the mid-1990s I was a big proponent of Dr. John Lee's natural progesterone treatment for osteoporosis. He reported a "case collection" of one hundred women who, after applying the progesterone cream (along with making basic dietary changes, exercising, and taking nutritional supplements) over a three-year period, had an average increase in bone density of 14 percent. This treatment plan made sense to me at the time, and I not only recommended it to my patients, I also followed it myself. In the longer term, however, because I owned and directed my own osteoporosis clinic I discovered that the protocol did not improve the bone density of those of us who tried it.

The fact is that there *are* progesterone receptors on osteoblasts (the cells that build bone); however, there are no studies showing that progesterone creams or pills can increase bone density anywhere near 14 percent in three years, and certainly not in postmenopausal women. Progesterone may benefit bone health—a topic about which you'll read more in the next chapter—but don't expect a progesterone supplement to result in a huge jump in bone density.

What's Going On with All the False Claims?

Over the years I've encountered numerous individuals and vendors who report increases in bone density based on the use of specific nutrients or supplements. I could share many more stories like the ones I've shared above. What's going on here? Is everyone who reports a gain in bone mass a charlatan? Or do these people actually believe what they're saying? I think that most people believe that what they're reporting is accurate.

So why do so many believe their bone density has increased when it has not? Earlier in the book we saw how the limitations inherent in bone density testing combined with errors made by untrained care providers could lead to false perceptions of changes in bone mass. As we learned in Chapter 2, the following are just some of the factors that account for these misperceptions:

o failure to use the same testing facility and same machine for all tests

o poor patient positioning (e.g., incorrect hip rotation can lead to test results that are off by as much as 7 percent)

o insufficient maintenance (not all testing facilities maintain their DXA machines in accordance with manufacturer guidelines)

o limited education (often, testing and/or reporting errors occur because the technicians and reporting doctors have no training in bone densitometry)

Don't lose heart; there is good news. Although bone-building isn't easy and there are no magic bullets, you *can* increase bone quality and possibly bone density—even as you grow older, when bone-building is most difficult. A good example would be an eighty-year-old woman who finds it hard to be physically active, and let's also imagine that she has gastrointestinal problems that are compounding her bone loss. Even at her age, she can positively impact the health of her bones if she is able to address her GI problems, because doing so will enable her to absorb more bone-building nutrients. As she improves her bone health, she also reduces her fracture risk. Ultimately, fracture prevention is the name of the game.

Studies have shown that a healthy, bone-supportive nutritional program and a robust exercise program can increase bone density and therefore reduce fracture risk. I have seen many of my own patients stop bone loss and gain bone density, but not easily. One of my post-menopausal patients experienced a gain in bone mass of 12 percent after a three-year lifestyle-change program that included rigorous exercise (including weight lifting), proper nutrition, and nutritional supplements. Another patient with early menopause and a vitamin D deficiency experienced a gain in bone mass of 8 percent after a three-year program that included vitamin D and bioidentical hormone supplementation and lifestyle changes. (You'll learn more about bone-healthy lifestyle choices in later chapters.)

Finally, in addition to the fact that it's possible to improve bone health even as a person ages, another piece of good news is this: Exaggerations about the success of certain alternative treatments do not necessarily mean that the treatments are completely ineffective. After all, there is a long way between complete reversal of osteoporosis and no help at all, so keep this in mind when evaluating claims. Most claims are founded on a grain of truth; that means many of these treatments may be beneficial for your bones, even if they're not miracle cures.

The next section describes some of the better-known alternative treatments that are said to reduce bone loss and increase bone density. Again, be aware that although most of the products discussed have some merit, and some are even backed by small studies suggesting they do help bone, none will "reverse" osteoporosis or increase bone density to any significant degree on their own. Still, these products may help your bones. They *may* improve the quality of your bones, and they *may* cause small increases in bone density. *The only thing I've found so far that can truly turn bone loss into bone growth amounts to a combination of permanent lifestyle changes and therapeutic interventions (sometimes medications, but always nutrition and exercise) that are appropriate given a patient's particular history and health status.*

If you have osteoporosis, remember that in order to choose the treatments that are right for you, you need to know which risk factors or secondary conditions might have contributed to your low bone density— for example, gastrointestinal problems, certain medications, or poor diet. You also need to know whether you are currently losing bone. As you've read in previous chapters, changes in bone density can be detected through a comparison of two bone density tests, if the tests are done correctly (see Chapters 2 and 3). But the best way to know if you are *actively* losing bone is through lab tests that evaluate bone turnover. Depending on your history and risk factors you may also need tests that can identify any secondary conditions (e.g., parathyroid disease, vitamin D deficiency, or kidney disease) that could result in bone loss (see Chapter 5). Finally, here's another tip to guide you in your search for alternative bone-building treatments: Any product that claims to (1) reverse osteoporosis or (2) increase bone density in a significant way, should be seriously questioned. Bone-building is a slow process, and, generally speaking, in order to determine if any loss or gain in bone density falls outside the 3 to 5 percent margin of error for DXA testing, comparison tests generally should be completed no earlier than two years after the initial test. (There are instances where bone loss is suspected to be high, in which case a bone density may be ordered before the two years. Such cases may include women who are going through menopause and patients with lab tests that indicate bone loss might be occurring.)

Alternative Bone-Building Treatments: An Overview

Although the bone-building impact of many of the treatments and therapies described below is often exaggerated, they may still help your bones.

Soy

Soy, a food many believe to be beneficial to bone health, is a rich source of isoflavones. Indeed, many isoflavones, also referred to as phytoestrogens, can mimic some of the effects of human estrogen and could therefore potentially have a positive impact on bone.

Some studies have shown that Japanese women have healthier bones and fewer fractures than American women. This finding has largely been attributed to the soy foods consumed by Japanese people.

In Japan, though, soy tends to be used in relatively small amounts. Furthermore, it's most often consumed as a whole (unprocessed) food, and much of it is fermented, which adds to its health benefit. Some Americans, in contrast, consume a lot of soy, and they do so in forms that are not typically used by the Japanese. American food companies include soy as an ingredient in many processed foods, and many American consumers eat soy cheeses, soy burgers, soy milk, and soy protein drinks. Soy-vey! Some Americans consume much more soy than their Japanese counterparts.

The take-home message is this: The research on the impact of soy on bone is mixed. Soy may help to protect bone in people who have eaten it over the course of their entire lives. That said, it would be very difficult to determine whether adopting a diet high in soy would lead to better bone health, because it's difficult to isolate the effects of soy alone. Along the same lines, it's difficult to compare the outcomes of the diets of different cultures, because different societies also have different lifestyle habits that interact with diet. Bottom line: If soy *does* influence bone health for Americans, the influence is probably small.

Ipriflavone

Ipriflavone (IP) is a synthetic isoflavone derived from the natural iso-flavones found in soy. It is available in the United States by prescription or over the counter in health food stores and online, and it is an approved treatment for osteoporosis in Japan and in many European countries.

As is the case with soy, though, while some studies suggest that IP may promote bone-building and reduce fractures, the research remains mixed. IP was linked to increased bone density of the forearm in one small study of one hundred women, for example, but other research, such as that conducted in 2010 by the Warsaw University of Life Sciences, finds no "cause and effect relationship between the consumption of ipriflavone and maintenance of bone mineral density in post-menopausal women." In fact, most of the IP studies are animal studies, and as is the case with research on other alternative treatments, studies of humans have been both small-scale and short-term.

Genistein

Genistein is an isoflavone that is derived primarily from soy. Many over-the-counter products include genistein as a bone-supportive element. Although studies of genistein are mixed, it does appear to reduce the activity of the cells that break down bone (osteoclasts) while stimulating activity of the cells that build bone (osteoblasts). Genistein also appears to reduce the negative impact of estrogen loss in postmenopausal women. Finally, some studies have shown that genistein may stimulate estrogen-sensitive breast cancer cells.

Fosteum

Fosteum, which is marketed as a "medical food" and requires a prescription, is a combination of genistein, zinc chelazome, and vitamin D-3. The Fosteum website claims that "it effectively balances and restores the normal metabolic processes involved in bone turnover." Please note that the manufacturer of this supplement warns that it should not be used by anyone at risk for reproductive cancer.

Certain Calcium Products

Several calcium supplements are said to impact bone density to a greater extent than other calcium products. These include:

Coral calcium: The claim for coral calcium goes something like this: Okinawa is home to significant expanses of coral reef, and people in Okinawa have fewer fractures and live into and beyond their nineties, so they must get a lot of coral calcium in their diet. There is no research to support this claim! Essentially, coral calcium supplements contain calcium carbonate and some trace minerals. Furthermore, the coral calcium in these products is harvested from dead coral, not living (because living coral reefs are endangered and therefore protected), and dead coral often contains pollutants that must be removed. Bottom line: I do not recommend this product.

Raw calcium: Raw calcium is advertised as superior because it is derived from algae sources. This product uses slick and clever marketing. At least one version boasts that it also contains "raw" vitamin D-3 and D-2 and other "raw" ingredients, and that it is gluten and dairy free. (Of course, there are no cows or wheat fields in the ocean.) Raw calcium is said to reduce one's risk for osteoporosis—a sly statement that is true, because (a) calcium is certainly essential to bone, (b) if you have a calcium deficiency, bone loss will occur, and (c) if you compensate for that deficiency, you'll likely reduce your risk of developing osteoporosis.

Raw calcium is probably very digestible and is likely a very good form of calcium. But there are no studies proving its superiority to other forms of calcium, and certainly no significant human studies showing that it increases bone density or reduces fracture risk.

Microcrystalline hydroxyapatite (MCHC): MCHC, which is derived from ground-up bovine (cow) bone, was developed based on the theory that humans can increase bone density if they ingest calcium in this form. The multiple studies that have examined this product are mostly small, and several are of questionable design. In 2009 a meta-analysis of six controlled trials found MCHC to be more effective than calcium carbonate in increasing bone density. Still, I remain unconvinced that this is a superior calcium source, in part because some bone products have been linked with heavy-metal contamination.

Lactoferrin

Lactoferrin is a protein found in milk. It appears to have a positive effect on bone turnover: Multiple animal studies have shown that it decreases bone resorption and increases bone formation. Lactoferrin supplements are said to pose no problems for those who are sensitive to dairy, so it may be a wise choice for some. If you want to try lactoferrin and are sensitive to dairy, be sure to discuss it with your treating doctor.

Milk Basic Protein

Milk basic protein (MBP) consists of high concentrations of several proteins found in whey, the liquid that remains after milk has been curdled and strained in the process of making cheese. Although studies on MBP are limited, there has been some research on three specific MBP proteins: lactoferrin, angiogenin, and cystatin C, each of which are thought to have a positive impact on bone density. Although the impact appears to be small, MBP is probably good for overall bone health.

Strontium Citrate

Like strontium ranelate, or Protelos, which you read about in Chapter 6, strontium citrate is a compound containing the element strontium. The research on strontium citrate is very limited. Whereas we do know that strontium *ranelate* has been shown to increase bone density and decrease fracture risk, we don't yet know whether strontium *citrate* will have the same impact on bone. What we do know is that strontium in any form ends up in the bone, replacing some of the calcium and remaining there, to some extent, for the duration of one's life. (We also know that any form of strontium will show false increases in bone density, but the extent of the false positives is unknown. I frequently see comments on the Internet advising people to ask the bone-testing facilities to account for these false increases in their calculations. But this is not possible. Currently we do not have a way to measure the false increase in bone density that results when you take a supplement or medication that includes strontium.)

Keep in mind that Protelos has side effects. This non–FDA approved drug is currently used to treat osteoporosis in Canada and Europe, but in April 2013 the European Medicines Agency confirmed the recommendation to restrict its use due to concerns about its link to adverse cardiac events. Read about the side effects of strontium ranelate before considering strontium citrate, and be aware that strontium citrate has not been fully studied. If you have serious osteoporosis and you simply will not entertain the idea of using conventional medications, then you may consider the benefits of this supplement to outweigh the risks. Even so, it's important to familiarize yourself with both forms of strontium before considering using it.

Herbal Remedies

Chinese herbs have been used for centuries, and some formulas are specifically created to support bone health. One of the more common Chinese preparations prescribed for osteoporosis is yin yang huo (also known as Herba Epimedii or HEP). In addition, Western herbs such as nettles and oat straw are loaded with bone-building nutrients. Though I am not aware of any research on Western herbs, there is some research that links HEP with a reduction in markers of bone turnover. In sum, herbal medicine may be helpful for bone. In Chapter 10 you will learn more about some of the best herbal supplements to include in your bone-health program.

Alternative Therapies

Although not all practitioners of alternative therapies are well-versed in the diagnostic tests needed to evaluate bone health, others are able to assess and treat patients with osteoporosis. Based on your reading of previous chapters, you now have some idea about what to expect from a doctor who's able to take the steps—and the time—needed to properly assess your case. Make sure that whoever oversees your osteoporosis treatment has a good understanding of lab tests and bone density testing.

A few of the therapies you may consider as you continue on your quest for bone health include:

Chiropractic: Chiropractic treatment is a system of "hands on" medicine that utilizes adjustments (manipulations) of fixations and/or misaligned joints, especially those in the spinal column. The entire body—including bones, muscles, and organs—is in some way under the direction of the nervous system. Chronic and acute nerve interference can impede the functioning of organs and the musculoskeletal system. Chiropractic doctors are trained to skillfully adjust (manipulate) the spine; some doctors also adjust other joints, including the extremities (arms and legs). If you have sustained a low-force fracture or if you have significant osteoporosis, consider seeing a chiropractor who offers nonforce techniques for adjusting the spine.

Acupuncture: Acupuncture treatment involves the insertion of specialized needles into the skin in order to stimulate certain points on the body. Described in terms of traditional Chinese medicine, acupuncture points lie along energy (chi) channels called "meridians," which are stimulated by acupuncture to balance the flow of chi throughout the body. Some acupuncturists also prescribe Chinese herbal combinations as well as rehabilitative exercises. Research has shown that acupuncture is effective as a pain reliever, and that it also increases blood flow. I am unaware of any studies showing that acupuncture impacts bone health; however, I personally believe that free-flowing chi is important for overall health, including the health of our bones.

Naturopathy: Naturopathy centers on the theory that diseases can be treated without resorting to drugs, using a wide range of natural techniques such as diet and exercise. Many naturopaths place a special emphasis on nutrition. Not surprisingly, naturopaths typically do not prescribe medications as part of their treatment protocols, although in some states they are permitted to prescribe some medications.

Note: Depending on state regulations, some chiropractors and naturopaths are able to order the diagnostic tests required to assess and monitor osteoporosis. Acupuncturists, unless they are a doctor of oriental medicine, are not licensed to order lab tests or bone density tests.

Vibration therapy: Vibration therapy involves the transmission of vibration to the body through contact areas such as the feet or buttocks. Vibration platforms are currently all the rage, and there are exercise centers that provide intense vibration therapy, but I have concerns about the safety of intense vibration, especially for elderly people. There is a type of vibration platform that I do recommend, however, and you'll learn more about it in Chapter 11.

Alternative Treatments Help Chronic Inflammation

Holistic practitioners tend to recommend treatments that help patients resolve inflammatory processes. This is good news, because as it turns out inflammation plays a significant role in many illnesses. Inflammation has been linked to diseases of the thyroid gland and gastrointestinal system—and also to active bone loss. It is beyond the scope of this chapter to fully explain inflammation and its impact on bone, but the take-home message is twofold: When active bone loss is occurring, an inflammatory process may be the culprit—and many of these conditions can resolve or be helped by alternative therapies through their focus on diet, GI health, and exercise.

Lab Tests to Verify Treatment Effectiveness

So, after taking into account your health history and the risk factors that impact your bone health, and after being tested to identify any secondary conditions that may be impacting your bones, you've decided upon a treatment or a combination of treatments. You know better than to expect a miracle, but how do you know if your program is helping you? You could always have a follow-up bone density test to see if there is an increase in bone density, but, generally speaking, you would need to allow two years between your initial test and a second one, and I don't recommend waiting that long. Instead, have your doctor repeat any lab tests that are suggestive of bone loss. Some of the repeat tests will show you whether a contributing problem such as vitamin D deficiency has been corrected. And it's very important to monitor markers of bone turnover (see Chapter 5). If bone resorption is high, repeat the bone marker tests in a few months to see whether the resorption has stabilized. Keep in mind that bone turnover tests are tricky. Bone markers vary from day to day, and they vary significantly, so there needs to be a high rate of change in order for the results to be accepted as "true." A 20 to 30 percent improvement is most likely a result you can trust.

Alternative Medicine: A Different Perspective

As I noted at the beginning of the chapter, many consumers use alternative bone-health remedies and hands-on treatments as a means to avoid the serious risks associated with osteoporosis medications. One of the great things about integrative doctors is that they pay attention to risk factors such as stress, inflammation, and other secondary health-related conditions that impact bone negatively. Along the same lines, they tend to take a much more active role in helping patients to make effective lifestyle changes.

In today's era of managed care, Western medicine gives a nod to what should be done, but integrative doctors typically spend more time with patients and focus much more on the lifestyle changes that promote health and healing. (In my first meeting with a patient, for example, I meet with him or her for ninety minutes, not fifteen.) In other words, integrative doctors tend to provide more than the boilerplate advice that patients often receive in the last five minutes of a conventional medical appointment ("Take Tums for added calcium, eat dairy three times a day and do weight-bearing exercise"). Some alternative doctors have patients keep a diary of important lifestyle habits such as exercise and diet—and then work with patients to change habits that aren't consistent with health and well-being. Health care that promotes true well-being goes beyond prescriptions that treat symptoms or lifestyle advice that's almost an afterthought. The most effective health-care practitioners will go that extra step, practicing in ways that truly motivate patients to take responsibility for their health.

Sometimes, reminders of the importance of lifestyle factors such as diet and exercise can be discouraging because habits take effort to develop and we don't expect to see immediate results when we do change our habits. The reality, though, is that even if the effects of these changes are relatively subtle, most of the time a genuine, sustained effort leads to positive, lasting results. The remaining chapters of this book are dedicated to giving you the information you need to adopt healthy habits that promote bone health.

 KEY POINTS FROM CHAPTER 7

o Integrative medicine is the best approach to preventing and treating osteoporosis.

o There are no "miracle" cures for osteoporosis.

o Be wary of claims that any single product will increase bone density.

o Many alternative therapies can help build healthy bone tissue at any age.

o Lifestyle, diet, and exercise must be the foundation of any bone-health program.

o Bone strength is determined by a combination of bone density and bone quality.

Hormones and
Your Bones

In the last chapter we saw how an integrative approach to health views the body as a complex system in which the well-being of any given part is impacted by the well-being and functioning of other parts. This chapter focuses on an area of major concern for integrative health-care providers who specialize in bone health and osteoporosis—namely, the many hormones that impact bone growth and bone maintenance. If you're working with an integrative doctor or other integrative health care professional, chances are he or she is going to talk to you about the state of your hormones.

Hormones: A Review

What are hormones, exactly? Hormones are naturally produced chemical "messengers" that are manufactured within various organs or glands and then secreted into the bloodstream so that their "messages" can be received by other parts of the body. Most hormones are produced by a group of glands known collectively as the endocrine system (see Figure 8.1). Endocrine glands are located in several parts of the body, but they are considered one system because of their similar functions and their relationship to each other.

How do hormones communicate their messages to other bodily systems? Clearly, any hormone that enters the bloodstream travels throughout the body, but only the cells that are sensitive to that par-

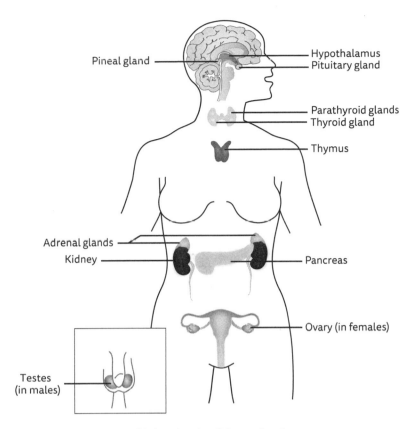

FIGURE 8.1. Major glands of the endocrine system

ticular hormone will respond to its chemical signal. Once the hormone attaches to these cells' "receptor" sites, the hormone essentially "flips a switch" in the body—a switch that may govern growth, development, or other mental and physical functions depending on the hormone in question. It makes sense, then, that the body's functioning is impaired when the hormones are not present at the levels they should be, or when cells for some reason fail to respond to the hormone's message the way they should.

In short, when each of the hormones is present in the right proportions, and when the receptor cells function as they should, body systems are stable. But hormones can be abnormally low, excessive, or absent, and when hormonal balance is lost, it causes problems in the body, resulting in symptoms that can range from unpleasant to severe. The symptoms of hormonal imbalance are many, and can include depression, anxiety, severe headaches, joint pain—and bone loss. A disruption in the balance of hormones produced by one gland or set of glands can cause other glandular systems to malfunction as well. Hormonal imbalance can be caused by a number of factors, including poor nutrition, stress, aging, blockages in "nerve flow" (i.e., distortions in the "flow" of the activity of the nerves), and even environmental toxins. Sadly, many people with hormone imbalances are put on symptom-focused medications when their symptoms—depression, for example—could be resolved with a treatment that corrects the underlying imbalance, benefitting the body as a whole.

It's essential to have the right amounts of hormones in the body in order for normal physiological functions to take place, including those that build and maintain bone. The purpose of this chapter is to give you an overview of some of the main hormones that impact bone growth and bone maintenance, namely, the growth hormones, calcium-regulating hormones, sex hormones, adrenal hormones, and thyroid hormones. Later in the chapter I'll share some of the ways you can balance hormones naturally, and we'll consider whether hormone-replacement therapy (HRT) or hormone therapy (HT) should be considered both for symptomatic relief and as a treatment to slow bone loss, especially at and after menopause for certain women. As we consider various hormone therapies, we'll take a brief look at the controversial area of bioidentical hormones versus nonbioidentical hormones.

Hormones That Affect Bone Health

This section describes the key hormonal players that can make or break bone health.

Growth Hormone and IGF-1

Growth hormone, also known as human growth hormone or somatotropin, stimulates cell regeneration and reproduction. The effects of growth hormone (GH) on the tissues of the body can generally be described as anabolic—that is, it builds tissue. The dramatic increase in height that occurs during childhood is the most widely known effect of GH. It also increases and helps maintain muscle mass. GH stimulates the production of insulin-like growth factor 1 (IGF-1), which in turn stimulates the cells that build bone (osteoblasts).

Growth hormone declines with aging. Symptoms of low GH in adults include reduced muscle mass and muscle strength, low bone mass or osteoporosis, increased body fat (especially around the waistline), and chronic inflammation. Low IGF-1 levels can lead to sarcopenia, or muscle wasting. Studies have shown that many people with severe osteoporosis, especially the elderly, have low IGF-1 blood levels, and many elderly people with osteoporosis also have severe sarcopenia.

The good news is that muscle-building exercise and deep sleep are two things that can increase GH, even in our later years, but only to a limited extent. Some doctors in the United States prescribe growth hormone for older patients as an antiaging substance. Although this use is legal, GH is a complex hormone about which much is still unknown—and that includes its safety as an antiaging supplement. If you have muscle wasting and/or osteoporosis, however, GH therapy may be a consideration. Testing for GH is difficult, but doctors can test for IGF-1 if a deficiency is suspected. Replacement of GH and IGF-1 may benefit bone and muscle health in those who are deficient in the hormones.

Calcium-Regulating Hormones

When it comes to bone, calcium tends to get a lot of attention, and for good reason. As much as 99 percent of the calcium in the body is stored in the bones. Bones serve as a reservoir for calcium, and they also play a major role in the maintenance of blood calcium levels, which must be kept within a relatively narrow range. Calcium is critical to many, if not most, of our body's various functions; for example, blood clotting, brain function, and muscle contractions, including heart contractions. Moreover, if we consistently have low blood calcium, the body will set in motion the release of calcium from the bones to carry out physical functions such as muscle contraction.

Blood calcium is regulated primarily by three hormones: parathyroid hormone (PTH), calcitonin, and calcitriol.

Parathyroid hormone: PTH is secreted by the four tiny parathyroid glands, which are located behind the thyroid (in the neck). PTH signals the osteoclasts to break down bone tissue, which increases calcium in the blood and stimulates the kidneys to reabsorb calcium.

Calcitonin: Calcitonin is secreted by the thyroid gland. In some ways it counteracts parathyroid hormone. When blood calcium is too high calcitonin decreases it by inhibiting osteoclast activity, inhibiting calcium absorption by the intestines, and acting on the kidneys to excrete calcium in the urine.

Calcitriol: This hormone, secreted by the kidneys, is the active form of vitamin D. It increases blood calcium levels by increasing calcium absorption from the small intestines and by increasing reabsorption of calcium by the kidneys. Through a circuitous route, it also stimulates osteoclasts to release calcium from the bone. Several studies utilizing bone biopsies have concluded that calcitriol does not increase bone formation.

As you can see, parathyroid hormone (PTH), calcitonin, and calcitriol assist the bones with their calcium-regulating functions by directly impacting the cells that build up or break down bone. The osteoclasts break down bone to release calcium into the blood when blood levels are too low. On the flip side, when blood levels of calcium are too high there are mechanisms in place to lower them. Sometimes, however, blood calcium levels get out of balance for some reason, remaining abnormally low or high, states referred to as "hypocalcemia" and "hypercalcemia," respectively. Both conditions can result in serious health consequences, and because the bones must compensate for problematic blood calcium levels, both low and high blood calcium can indicate the occurrence of bone loss.

Hypocalcemia (insufficient blood calcium) is commonly caused by low calcium intake or gastrointestinal problems that lead to calcium malabsorption. Secondary hyperparathyroidism (overactivity of the parathyroid gland, resulting in too much PTH), which can be caused by a vitamin D deficiency, can also result in low blood calcium levels. Vitamin D deficiencies can result from kidney disease, lack of sun exposure, or low vitamin D intake.

Hypercalcemia (elevated blood calcium) can be caused by a pituitary tumor (primary hyperparathyroidism). The tumor (most often benign) produces excess parathyroid hormone that breaks down bone and typically results in elevated blood calcium levels. Elevated calcium can also signal the presence of multiple myeloma (a type of bone cancer) or other cancers.

As you can see, the calcium-regulating hormones play a significant role in our bone health. It is critical that your primary health-care provider properly understand the relationship between these hormones and bone, especially if you have been diagnosed with osteoporosis. An appreciation of the importance of the calcium-regulating hormones will guide your doctor in ordering tests that can identify any calcium-maintenance problems. If it has been determined that you have too much or too little calcium in your blood, additional tests should be ordered to figure out why. Patients with osteoporosis should have their calcium, PTH, and vitamin D tested. Remember, it isn't just high or low results that signal a problem; "high-normal" and "low-normal" results are also red flags. See Chapter 5 for more information on the tests that can help you monitor your calcium levels.

Sex Hormones

The sex hormones, too, have a direct impact on bone. Estrogen, for example, keeps osteoclasts in check; it also stimulates osteoblasts to some extent. That's why, at menopause, women can lose a lot of bone; the loss of estrogen means a decrease in osteoclast inhibition.

All of us need well-functioning sex hormones for good bones. And all of us produce both male and female sex hormones, including the androgens (testosterone and DHEA), estrogens, and progesterone. The androgens are considered "male" because they have masculinizing effects, while estrogens have feminizing effects—so although both types are present in each sex, men and women differ in their levels of each type. Both male and female sex hormones play a major role in our lifetime accrual of bone mass, especially during adolescence, and also later in life, when we're primarily maintaining the bone we have.

Generally speaking, as we age, the impact of the sex hormones on bone health is much greater for women than for men—mainly because women experience a significant drop in certain hormone levels once they hit menopause. Males also experience age-related decreases in sex hormones, which does impact their bones, but women are at a much higher risk for bone loss, and at an earlier age. Women can lose 20 percent or more of their bone mass in the years just before and after menopause. The rest of this section describes the impact of the sex hormones on women and men, with an emphasis on women.

Women and Their Sex Hormones

The female sex hormones—the estrogens and progesterone—as well as some testosterone are produced primarily in the ovaries. These hormones interact to coordinate a woman's menstrual cycle during her reproductive years.

Estrogen: Women's bodies produce over twenty types of estrogen, the main ones being estrone, estradiol, and estriol.

- *Estrone (E1)*: Estrone is the main estrogen a woman's body manufactures following menopause, at which time its production shifts from the ovaries to predominantly the adipose (fat cells) tissue. As the ovaries age and the production of estradiol decreases, estrone becomes the dominant estrogen, yet it remains at a low level, so its impact on bone tissue is minimal.

- *Estradiol (E2)*: Estradiol, the most potent of the estrogens, is the primary hormone produced by the ovaries prior to menopause. Estradiol inhibits osteoclastic activity, and, to a small extent, also stimulates the osteoblasts. During a woman's reproductive years (including adolescence), estradiol is the dominant bone-building estrogen. Estradiol levels fluctuate with the menstrual cycle from low to very high during reproductive years. After menopause estradiol drops to a low level and stays there.

- *Estriol (E3)*: Known as "the pregnancy estrogen," estriol has a minimal impact on bone. It has a limited effect on osteoclasts and occurs in significant amounts only during pregnancy, when it is produced by the placenta. Estriol is the weakest of the three estrogens and thought by some to be a safer alternative for treating symptoms of menopause.

During the reproductive years, as mentioned above, most of the estrogen a woman produces is manufactured in the ovaries. However, body fat also produces estrogen (estrone). Overproduction of estrogen can be a problem when women carry too much fat at any age. On the other hand, for various reasons, very thin women may produce extremely low levels of estradiol and estrone. This is one reason why estrogen therapy is an important consideration for certain women, especially if they have osteoporosis. Estrogen levels should always be checked around the time of menopause for women with risk factors for developing osteoporosis (see Chapter 4 for risk factors).

Progesterone: Most of the progesterone produced by women's bodies occurs in response to ovulation, once the egg is ejected from the ovaries. Progesterone (think "pro-gestation") readies the uterine lining for pregnancy, allowing a fertilized egg to attach to the uterine wall for further development. No ovulation, no progesterone—which is particularly relevant to young women who have anovulatory cycles (menstrual cycles without egg production), as studies have shown that numerous anovulatory cycles can result in bone loss. A range of conditions, including pituitary dysfunction, ovarian dysfunction, hypothyroidism, and nutritional deficiencies, can cause anovulation.

Osteoblast cells have progesterone receptors, and some research shows that, for younger women, low progesterone can lead to bone loss. Progesterone therapy has not been shown to be effective in building bone in postmenopausal women; however, researcher Jerilynn Prior concludes that progesterone prevents bone loss in pre- and possibly perimenopausal women. Progesterone therapy should also be considered as a way to balance a woman's hormones, especially before menopause, when ovulation and progesterone production are erratic.

Testosterone: Most testosterone in women is produced in the ovaries, although some is manufactured in the adrenal glands. Testosterone plays a role in sexual desire and the development of muscle mass. In terms of testosterone's impact on bone, for women it occurs primarily during adolescence. It's also likely that testosterone supports bone maintenance in postmenopausal women, perhaps because it can metabolize to estrogen.

Imbalances in Women's Sex Hormones

What happens when a woman's sex hormones are out of balance? Imbalances in estrogen and progesterone can occur at any age but are most common during puberty, before menopause, and for many years after menopause. Women can also suffer from low testosterone, experiencing symptoms that include low libido, muscle weakness, and others that may resemble those associated with hypothyroidism. Symptoms associated with sex hormone imbalances in women include:

- bone loss
- depression
- irregular periods
- memory lapses
- acne
- heart palpitations
- thinning skin
- night sweats
- sleep disturbances
- vaginal dryness
- increased body/facial hair
- foggy thinking
- uterine fibroids
- thyroid dysfunction

- loss of muscle mass
- hot flashes
- low libido
- mood swings (PMS)
- headaches
- fibrocystic breasts
- nervousness
- poor concentration
- urinary incontinence
- weight gain
- cystic ovaries
- irritability
- polycystic ovarian syndrome
- heavy menses and menstrual irregularities

PMS, Hysterectomy, and Early Menopause Can Be Bad for the Bones

To recap: In women, the female sex hormones are crucial for bone and are produced (1) primarily in the ovaries, (2) during a woman's reproductive years, and (3) when a woman is ovulating. Stated another (somewhat oversimplified) way: In women, robust levels of bone-building sex hormones are all about the healthy—and reproductive—functioning of the ovaries. That is why menopause and irregular menstruation can have such a significant negative impact on women's bone health. Let's look at some events that can interfere with the production of the sex hormones that are crucial to bone health in women.

- PMS: Although some PMS (premenstrual syndrome) symptoms can be normal, severe symptoms are *not* normal. Both severe PMS and irregular menstruation are indicative of hormonal imbalances that can lead to bone loss. Remember, women's ability to build bone is severely restricted during months when they fail to menstruate. If you have severe PMS symptoms or your periods are irregular, I encourage you to see your gynecologist for a physical examination to make sure your female organs are healthy. You may also want to see someone who specializes in hormone balancing (using bioidentical hormones when appropriate—see below). Also, keep in mind that most PMS symptoms will resolve with proper nutritional support and exercise.

- Hysterectomy with ovary removal: Not too long ago, conventional medical wisdom held that women who were not going to continue having children would be better off having their ovaries removed so as to eliminate their (small) risk for ovarian cancer. But a woman's ovaries continue to benefit her bones, even after she's stopped menstruating. We learned earlier that estradiol, the most potent of the estrogens, drops significantly after menopause, but the ovaries continue to produce a small amount of both estradiol and testosterone long after menopause—so the ovaries continue to benefit bone throughout the female lifespan. A hysterectomy should be considered only as a last resort, but if you end up deciding to have surgery, keep your ovaries if you can!

- Early menopause: The average age of menopause is fifty-two. (The definitive marker of menopause is when menstruation has ceased for one year.) A significantly early menopause can have a devastating impact on bone if the hormones that are no

(cont'd.)

longer being produced are not replaced. If you stop menstruating in your forties (or earlier), make sure to have your hormones tested. Early menopause is a true indication for hormone replacement therapy, a topic that's discussed later in the chapter.

Men and Their Sex Hormones

Testosterone: As stated earlier, men produce many of the same sex hormones that women do, including the so-called female sex hormones. For men, the sex hormone with the greatest impact on bone is testosterone. Most testosterone in men is produced in the testicles, though some is also produced in the adrenal glands. Men's testosterone levels are about seven times higher than those in women.

We learned that for women a drastic change takes place at menopause that lowers hormone levels, resulting in significant bone loss for some. Men don't go through such an extreme drop in their hormones; rather they experience a slower, more gradual loss. "Andropause" is the term for the hormone loss—primarily a drop in testosterone—that occurs in men as they age, usually beginning in their sixties.

Testosterone deficiency is the number-one cause of osteoporosis in men. Younger men can have this condition and should be checked if they have osteoporosis or symptoms of hormone imbalance. Signs of testosterone deficiency in men include reduced libido, erectile dysfunction, hot flushes, sweats, breast tenderness, depressed mood or irritability, poor concentration and memory problems, sleep disturbances, increased body fat, fatigue, reduced muscle mass and strength—and low bone density and osteoporosis.

There is a concern that testosterone therapy could increase the risk of testicular cancer in some men. For this reason, testosterone therapy is primarily recommended for men who have low testosterone levels, hypogonadism, or erectile dysfunction.

Estrogen: Men produce estrogens, too. In addition, testosterone metabolizes to estrogen. It is unknown whether testosterone itself, or the fact that it metabolizes to estrogen, is what primarily protects bone in men as they age. As with women, if men carry a lot of extra fat they produce more estrogen.

Progesterone: The bulk of progesterone that men produce is from the adrenal glands. For men, the effects of progesterone on bone are thought to be minimal.

Adrenal Hormones

Some of the hormones that are often categorized as adrenal hormones are also important for bone. The adrenal glands, located on top of the kidneys, produce some of the same sex hormones as those produced by the testes and ovaries. In both men and women the adrenals produce small amounts of estrogen and testosterone. They also produce several other hormones that have a direct or indirect impact on the bones, including DHEA, androstenedione, aldosterone, and the stress hormones cortisol and adrenaline. When the adrenal hormones are imbalanced, especially as a result of prolonged stress, the impact on the bones can be significant. The subsections below focus on two of the most important adrenal hormones, DHEA and cortisol.

DHEA (dehydroepiandrosterone): Popularly known as an antiaging hormone, DHEA in supplement form is strongly touted by doctors who promote antiaging. Whereas stress, diet, and lifestyle all contribute to the amount of DHEA the body can produce, the hormone is at its highest level in people in their twenties. DHEA levels begin to decline after the age of thirty or so, and most people, especially women, produce much lower levels once they reach fifty.

The impact of DHEA on bone has not been well researched; however, we do know that it converts to testosterone and estrogen in both men and women and therefore probably impacts bone positively. When DHEA supplementation is used appropriately, it can play a key role in hormone balancing, which might also benefit the bones to some extent.

A word of caution: DHEA supplements are readily available without a prescription at health food stores and pharmacies. It is advertised mostly as a weight-loss supplement, and bodybuilders also use it to boost muscle growth. It is not wise to take this supplement without the guidance of a health practitioner who will evaluate you on an individual basis, assessing your complete hormone status before determining if DHEA is right for you.

Cortisol: All of us experience stress as a normal part of daily life, and when we do our adrenal glands secrete cortisol, which has been dubbed the "stress hormone." Cortisol, formerly known as hydrocortisone, regulates our body's fight-or-flight response to stress, enabling us to respond and adapt to life's daily challenges. It also reduces inflammation in the body and assists with the functioning of the immune system. An excess, long-term exposure to cortisol—brought about by prolonged stress—reduces calcium absorption in the intestines and can inhibit the bone-building cells, osteoblasts. This scenario can result in bone loss.

 Adrenal Imbalances

Imbalance of the adrenal hormones is one of the most common conditions I see in my practice. The typical cause is chronic stress, which can result in diminished adrenal function (sometimes called "adrenal exhaustion" or "adrenal fatigue") and may include the depletion of DHEA. DHEA and cortisol levels are most reliably determined using saliva tests. It takes time to resolve adrenal depletion, which is a condition that typically brews for months, if not years. You can promote adrenal balance by attending to the basics: Learn stress-management techniques, drink plenty of water, and regulate your blood sugar levels by eating small meals throughout the day. Along with potential bone loss, some of the most common symptoms of adrenal imbalance are listed below:

- allergies/asthma
- chemical sensitivities
- high blood sugar
- increased abdominal fat
- sleep disturbances
- autoimmune illness
- aches and pains
- chronic illness
- depression or anxiety

- arthritis
- morning/evening fatigue
- inflammation
- memory lapses
- susceptibility to infections
- sugar cravings
- infertility
- elevated triglycerides
- nervousness or irritability

Thyroid Hormones

The thyroid hormones—produced by the thyroid gland, located in the front of the neck—are the last but not least major category of hormones that have a direct impact on bone. As discussed above, the thyroid produces calcitonin, an important calcium-regulating hormone. It also manufactures other significant hormones: triiodothyronine (T3) and thyroxin (T4). T3 and T4 secretions are regulated by thyroid-stimulating hormone (TSH), which is produced by the pituitary gland. The thyroid hormones control growth and metabolism and provide energy, thus impacting the function of many systems in the body.

The thyroid gland can be overactive, a condition referred to as "hyperthyroidism," or underactive, known as "hypothyroidism," which is much more common. Hypothyroidism is most typically indicated by an elevated level of TSH. However, TSH can be normal yet T3 and/or T4 may be low, which can also indicate low thyroid function. Conversely, a very low TSH and an elevated T4 can point to hyperthyroidism. Not surprisingly, given the impact of these hormones on growth and metabolism, too much or too little of any of them can result in poor health generally—and potentially bone loss, too.

Hypothyroidism

As mentioned above, the most common thyroid imbalance is hypothyroidism (underactive thyroid hormone output), which is usually caused by thyroiditis (Hashimoto's disease), an autoimmune disease. Hypothyroidism is nine times more common in women than in men. It is interesting to note that women most often develop this condition during puberty, pregnancy, perimenopause, or menopause—all times when a woman's hormones are erratic. However, men, too, can suffer from hypothyroidism, and because it is less common in men, the diagnosis is often missed. Hashimoto's disease is diagnosed using thyroid antibody tests and sometimes an ultrasound test of the thyroid gland. (But hypothyroidism can also be present when antibody tests are normal.)

In recent years research has shown a connection between hypothyroidism and bone loss. Symptoms of low thyroid function include:

- dry, brittle hair and nails
- hair loss
- dry skin
- low body temperature, cold hands and feet
- elevated cholesterol
- constipation
- depression
- "brain fog"
- fatigue
- infertility
- low libido
- weight gain/inability to lose weight
- anxiety
- menstrual disturbances
- headaches
- joint and muscle pain

Some patients experience many of the symptoms of hypothyroidism, yet their TSH, T3, and T4 levels fall within normal limits. Recall from Chapter 5 that one can have lab results that barely fall within the normal limits while still experiencing significant symptoms. If that's true for you, your doctor needs to really pay attention to your symptoms for a more accurate diagnosis.

If you have hypothyroidism, do you need to take medications? Not necessarily. Many patients, especially borderline hypothyroid patients, do fine with a healthy dietary plan and nutritional support for optimal thyroid function. When it is necessary to take thyroid hormones there are several options to consider. For a website and books that provide information regarding the diagnosis and treatment of thyroid conditions, see Resources.

When it comes to bone health, you should be monitored if you're taking a thyroid medication. There is research showing a direct link between taking thyroid medications and bone loss. Many doctors today feel that if thyroid functioning is managed correctly, the patient's symptoms should be minimal and medications should not cause bone loss.

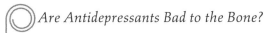

Are Antidepressants Bad to the Bone?

Anxiety and irritability, depression, "brain fog." When you consider some of the symptoms of thyroid or sex hormone imbalances, you see that they can impact not only one's physical condition but also one's mental functioning and mood. Unfortunately, hormone-related diagnoses are often "missed" by doctors, which means that many patients with hormone conditions are put on antidepressants. This may be problematic as some studies have linked bone loss to SSRIs (selective serotonin reuptake inhibitors), including widely used antidepressants such as Prozac and Zoloft. If you have mood symptoms such as anxiety or depression, be careful. You may want to consult with a provider who's well-versed in hormones, as hormone imbalances often have causes that can be corrected using natural means—for example, proper nutrition and exercise—benefitting both your mood and your bones.

Hyperthyroidism

Hyperthyroidism is the opposite of hypothyroidism; due to overactivity of the thyroid gland, the functioning of the body's systems is accelerated rather than slowed. While the most common cause of hyperthyroidism is thyrotoxicosis, an autoimmune condition known as Grave's disease, it can also be caused by an excess of thyroid medication. Low levels of TSH and elevated levels of T4 typically indicate hyperthyroidism.

Although less common than hypothyroidism, hyperthyroidism is strongly linked to bone loss. For some, symptoms such as agitation and anxiety may serve as a clue that the thyroid gland is overactive. Other common symptoms of hyperthyroidism include:

- insomnia
- diarrhea
- increased appetite
- rapid heartbeat/heart palpitations
- fatigue/muscle weakness
- sweating
- hair loss
- weight loss

What Causes Hormone Irregularities?

The material above lists some of the most common problems that can occur when hormones are out of balance—including, of course, bone loss. But what causes these imbalances?

There is a broad range of factors that cause hormonal irregularities, including certain health conditions—for example, tumors in the pituitary gland. Other factors are lifestyle-related, including smoking, insufficient water intake, poor dietary choices, and lack of exercise. This section provides a brief overview of some of the factors that are most strongly associated with hormone imbalances or insufficiencies.

Aging

Sex hormone levels decrease with aging in both men and women. As stated earlier, women can lose 20 percent or more of their bone density in the five- to ten-year period surrounding menopause. However, this loss does not have to occur. I do not consider it "normal" to lose bone. During the menopausal years it is especially important to hone your bone-building skills, as outlined in the chapters that follow.

Genetics

Many hormone-related conditions run in families. Thyroid disease, primary hyperparathyroidism, endometriosis, and early menopause are examples of hormone-related conditions that can have a genetic component. Having a genetic predisposition does not necessarily mean you will express the disease. Heart disease is a good example. If people eat a diet that does not support heart health, they may wind up with abnormal blood lipid (cholesterol) profiles, inflammation, and excess body weight, which predisposes them to heart disease, especially if they also have a genetic susceptibility.

GI Problems and/or Stress

Chronic emotional and/or physical distress and chronic gastrointestinal problems that cause nutritional deficiencies are other factors that can result in hormone imbalances. Quite often, these kinds of contributing factors can be corrected with lifestyle changes. As an example, I discovered that one of my patients had celiac disease (gluten intolerance; see Chapter 9) in the course of my assessment of her lab work. This forty five-year-old patient also had severe PMS and active bone loss, but once she adopted a healthy, gluten-free diet, her PMS disappeared. In addition, her bone loss stabilized.

Nutrition

As you will learn in Chapters 9 and 10, good bone health ultimately depends on good nutrition and a gastrointestinal system that can readily absorb nutrients. Like your bones, your endocrine system requires a constant supply of nutrients. Protein, certain fatty acids, and vitamin D are just a few examples of nutrients that are absolutely essential for hormone balance and, thus, healthy bones. Your hormone levels will suffer if your body isn't getting the nutrition it needs.

A Matter of Diet: Sophia's Story

Thirty-five-year-old Sophia came to my office to address her chronic depression and difficulty sleeping. She was also concerned because her depression symptoms increased around the time of her menstrual cycle. Sophia suspected that she suffered from hormone imbalances, but after reviewing her diet diary I noted that she did not eat much food during the day, and I knew that she was not getting the calories and nutrients she needed to fuel her body properly. Because her predominant mood state could have been caused by poor nutrition and sleep deficits (she had a four-year-old child), I elected not to order lab tests right away but instead started her on a nutrient-dense diet, asking her to eat three meals and two healthy snacks each day. Sophia increased her protein intake to account for 30 percent of her diet, and she added vitamin supplements, including a multiple vitamin, vitamin D, and fish oil. I also had her take extra vitamin C (500 mg four times a day) to help bolster her adrenal glands, which require vitamin C to function properly. She was also willing to eliminate processed carbohydrates and sugar. After one month Sophia's dietary program improved her symptoms of depression and insomnia by 80 percent!

Anorexia Nervosa

"Anorexia nervosa" is an eating disorder characterized by an unwillingness to maintain a normal body weight for age and height; in many cases it results in extreme weight loss. Although anorexia nervosa (often referred to as simply "anorexia") can occur at any age and in both sexes, it is most commonly seen in people in their teens and early twenties, especially girls and young women. Anorexia leads directly to inadequate nutritional intake, which over time results in weight loss and hormone depletion. Malnutrition and insufficient body fat can cause some girls to stop menstruating, and as we learned earlier bone loss occurs when menstruation stops or is irregular over a period of time.

Lack of Exercise

As you'll learn in Chapter 11, exercise is critical for bone health—and it's also good for the hormones. Multiple studies confirm that regular exercise can resolve mild to moderate hormone imbalances, in turn resolving symptoms such as depression, anxiety, and menstrual irregularities.

Exposure to Endocrine-Disrupting Chemicals

A wide variety of environmental chemicals can disrupt the endocrine system, many of them by exhibiting an abnormal estrogenic activity. Estrogenic "endocrine disruptors" can attach to the estrogen-receptor sites in any animal that has estrogen receptors—including humans. Estrogenic chemicals are found in many of the pesticides used in agriculture, in cleaning products, and in personal care products, including some preservatives (parabens) and sunscreen chemicals.

In today's world, most if not all of us are exposed to environmental endocrine disruptors on a routine basis. We know that when large amounts of such chemicals have been released into the environment, wildlife suffers from reproductive cancers and loss of reproductive ability. Most environmental scientists are concerned about the continued use of these chemicals and view them as hazardous to the environment and to the human body. Visit the website for the Environmental Working Group (www.EWG.org) for information about hazardous consumer and cleaning products.

Should You Consider Hormone Therapy?

Both men and women may be faced with recommendations of hormone therapy, and each individual needs to weigh the risks and benefits against his or her specific needs. What if, after reading about some of the most significant symptoms and causes of hormonal imbalance, you suspect you have a hormone condition? You now know that some hormone irregularities can be corrected with lifestyle changes such as reduced stress or modified diet—but what about hormone therapy? After all, if the problem is insufficient hormone levels, why not just add the hormones you need?

I'm a huge proponent of natural interventions, so I'd rather see you correct your hormone imbalances with lifestyle changes, if possible. The younger you are the more feasible it is to do so. However, for many, making such changes will simply not be enough to protect bone or, in some cases, to make up for bone loss that may have occurred after years of poor lifestyle choices.

Although many women with osteoporosis may benefit from hormone therapy, hormone replacement is especially important to consider for women entering an early menopause. Early menopause indicates a true need for hormone *replacement* therapy (HRT), especially in a woman in her twenties, thirties, or early forties. (The average age for menopause is fifty-two.) The same applies for men; younger men with low testosterone (hypogonadism) should also consider HRT.

I am a proponent of hormone therapies that use *bioidentical* hormones (see below) when doing so is appropriate; however, for women with estrogen-positive breast cancer, even bioidentical estrogen is not recommended by most doctors. For women who are entering menopause and who have low bone mass or osteoporosis, hormone therapy is a reasonable consideration. Studies have shown that estradiol can help minimize bone loss during the five to ten years postmenopause. Some doctors use estriol for symptomatic relief; however, estriol's impact on bone is minimal. Progesterone and testosterone are also used in some treatment protocols.

Some antiaging doctors prescribe high doses of hormones to mimic the levels we had in our youth. I generally do not agree with high-dose regimens for postmenopausal women or aging men. Instead, I prefer smaller amounts, just enough to quell symptoms and slow down bone loss. (Many books have been devoted to hormone balancing. See the Resources for some suggested titles on this topic.)

The rest of this section considers various questions relating to hormone therapy.

What Is the Best Way to Test for Hormone Levels?

Blood, urine, and saliva tests can be used to measure sex hormones and adrenal hormones (DHEA and cortisol). Thyroid hormones can only be tested through blood and urine. While there are differing opinions about each of these testing modalities, they each have their benefits. I typically use a combination of blood and saliva testing. You'll find a list of labs that can test your hormone levels in Resources. In addition to the lab work, your health-care practitioner will need to carefully assess your symptoms, because hormone levels change from day to day or even month to month for a variety of reasons and often do not provide an accurate diagnosis.

Are There Other Hormones That May Need to Be Tested?

Other hormones may need to be tested, especially if there is a possibility of hypogonadism in men or women. Some of the hormones that might be tested include pituitary hormones, luteinizing hormone (LH), follicle-stimulating hormone (FSH), adrenocorticotropic hormone (ACTH), and prolactin. Some prohormones (hormone precursors), such as pregnenolone, may also need to be tested. It is important to consider testing some of these hormones when significant symptoms arise.

Aren't There Risks Associated with the Use of Estrogen Replacement?

One of the main concerns about estrogen replacement therapy is that it may increase one's risk for breast cancer, strokes, or heart disease. Studies go back and forth as to whether or not the risks associated with estrogen replacement outweigh the benefits, but some research suggests that the benefits are worth it for most women who are candidates. In 2012 one major, much anticipated, and well-designed study (the KEEPS trial) shed a great deal of light on the safety of early hormone intervention. It looked at the impact of estrogen and progesterone therapy in postmenopausal women. Researchers stated that study outcomes "should provide reassurance to women who are recently menopausal and taking hormone therapy for short-term treatment of menopausal symptoms." The trial, which involved more than seven hundred women, found that estrogen/progesterone treatment obtained soon after menopause "appears to be safe; relieves many of the symptoms of menopause; and improves mood, bone density, and several markers of cardiovascular risk." One notable aspect of this study is that it included bioidentical estradiol and progesterone and did not rely exclusively on the equine hormone Premarin. Most studies in the past did not include bioidentical hormones. (For more information about bioidentical hormones, see the very next subsection. For more information about the KEEPS trial, visit www.menopause.org.)

What about long-term hormone therapy? Long-term use is a controversial issue you will need to consider carefully. Those who may benefit most are women who have osteoporosis and have very low body fat.

Bioidentical Hormones Versus Nonbioidentical Hormones?

If you've done any research on the topic of hormones, chances are you've run across the term "bioidentical." A particularly helpful description of BH comes from the Harvard Medical School: "The interest in a more natural approach to hormone therapy has focused attention on bioidentical hormones—hormones that are identical in molecular structure to the hormones women make in their bodies. They're not found in this form in nature but are made, or synthesized, from a plant chemical extracted from yams and soy. Bioidentical hormone therapy is often called 'natural hormone therapy' because bioidentical hormones act in the body just like the hormones we produce. But here again, that tricky word *natural* muddies the waters. Pregnant mares' urine is natural, but Premarin is not bioidentical, at least not to human estrogen. The same goes for Cenestin, which is made from plants but is not bioidentical."

Proponents of BH feel strongly that if hormone therapy is needed for hormone balancing, BH should be the first choice. Conventional doctors, on the other hand, most often recommend Premarin and Provera, both of which are nonbioidentical. This is a highly controversial subject, so make sure you learn enough about your hormone situation to make an informed choice, and that includes understanding the state of your bone health. All of the sex hormones can be produced as bioidentical hormones, and, in general, people tend to respond more favorably to BH therapy. Nonbioidentical hormones act on the body in ways that are different from the effects of bioidentical hormones. In addition, some of the effects of nonbioidentical hormones are undesirable; for example, nonbioidentical progesterone may cause depression, while bioidentical progesterone can act as a natural antidepressant.

I personally feel that Premarin should be taken off the market. Quite simply it is not the best estrogen for humans to take, and it is unnecessary for horses to be subject to having to provide urine for hormone treatment. Female horses must be made pregnant and kept in small quarters so their urine can be collected. Many are repeatedly impregnated for this purpose. We can debate whether the conditions for these horses are good or bad, but the additional point is this: Premarin is not even the best estrogen to use, period.

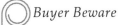 *Buyer Beware*

You can purchase progesterone creams and DHEA supplements online and in health food stores, but I do not recommend using either of these powerful hormones without guidance from a health care professional. I've had some patients whose hormone imbalances were made worse with these supplements.

Balancing Hormones Naturally

So you've read about the symptoms of hormonal imbalance, you suspect that you may have a hormonal irregularity, and, if possible, you'd like to avoid hormone replacement. What can you do to balance your hormones naturally, and will doing so suffice if you have been diagnosed with osteoporosis?

The following three chapters provide an excellent guide that can help you ensure that your body gets what it needs for proper hormone function and bone health. If your symptoms are only mild or moderate, upgrading your nutritional intake and increasing your physical activity may be all you need to do to adjust your hormone levels. If you have a significant hormone imbalance that requires HT, I strongly recommend that you consider working with a health-care provider who specializes in hormone balancing and is familiar with bioidentical hormones.

In Chapter 10 you will learn about what constitutes a bone-building diet—from proteins and fats to specific micronutrients. For the most part, the same nutrients are needed to balance sex hormones, thyroid hormones, and adrenal hormones. You will read about vitamins D, C, and A, the minerals calcium, magnesium, and zinc, and the healthy omega-3 fatty acids (available through sources such as fish oil, flax seeds, borage seeds, and seaweed). In addition, exercise and a healthy GI tract are especially important for sex hormone balance and for healthy thyroid and adrenal functions. One of the most important things you can do to stabilize your hormones is to eat regular meals, balance your macronutrients, and maintain healthy and consistent blood sugar levels by consuming small meals instead of large ones.

When the body's hormones are in balance they work together in harmony—and the bones benefit immensely. Our hormonal system is extremely complex, and even small imbalances can have a significant impact. The good news is this: Many hormone irregularities can be corrected with careful nutrition and plenty of exercise. You'll go a long way toward maximizing your hormone health if you follow the advice in the remainder of this book. In the next chapter, on digestion, you will learn how the bones depend on a healthy gastrointestinal tract that's able to absorb the nutrients you take in. Clearly, that information applies to your hormones as well.

 KEY POINTS FROM CHAPTER 8

o Calcium regulation is controlled by several hormones.

o Hormone balance is important throughout life for healthy bones.

(cont'd.)

o Hormones can often be balanced naturally with diet and digestive help.

o Women can lose up to 20 percent of their bone mass in the years following menopause.

o An excess of stress hormones can result in bone loss.

o To help minimize bone loss during the perimenopausal and postmenopausal years, bioidentical hormones should definitely be a consideration for women at risk for osteoporosis.

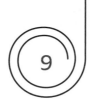

9

Getting a Gut Feeling about Your Bone Health

Osteoporosis is referred to as a "silent" disease because it comes on gradually rather than overnight and often surprises people by making itself known quite suddenly in the form of a broken bone. That said, the body can provide certain clues to suggest that you might be a candidate for bone loss, one of the most important of which is recurring digestive issues. Whether you're twenty or seventy, if you have regular digestive symptoms your body might be telling you that it's not getting what it needs, including what it needs to build and maintain bone.

In real estate, it's often said that what matters most is location, location, location. When it comes to bone health, what matters most is digestion, digestion, digestion. Although it's common to focus on one nutrient—calcium—when thinking about bone health, the fact is the bones need many nutrients, and the digestive system must be in good working order for them to receive the ones they need.

Bones are not dried-up, unchanging items, like a piece of sunbaked skeleton you might find while walking in the desert. As discussed in Chapter 1, they comprise a dynamic system with a rich blood supply and specialized cells that are in charge of replacing older, worn-out bone tissue with healthy new bone. To do this, the cells need a constant source of bone-building nutrients, including protein; minerals such as calcium, magnesium, phosphorus, and boron; and bone-essential vitamins such as A, D, K, and others. In order to get these vital nutrients to the bones, your digestive system needs to be able to break down and absorb the foods you eat. The quality of the food you consume is important as well. Your skeletal system needs nutrient-rich foods that will build and maintain healthy bone tissue rather than processed foods devoid of essential nutrients.

The body operates much like an orchestra. Different components come together, like instruments, to create a greater whole. Any single instrument or section that is out of tune will adversely affect the larger entity. Along the same lines, if your gut is out of tune, your bones and other organs will suffer over time.

A Trio of Related Conditions: My Story

I discovered firsthand how digestion was impacting my bones and my overall health when I hit menopause. Though I have always had food sensitivities, I discovered that by only occasionally eating the foods that gave me trouble, I could manage the symptoms, which included sinus congestion and an occasional skin rash. However, as my hormone levels began to decline as a natural result of aging, my reaction to the "problem" foods increased. The combination of irritating foods, hormonal changes, and the everyday stresses of life erupted into a major skin condition, with a new, more complicated itchy and painful rash around my mouth and nose. My dermatologist diagnosed me with perioral dermatitis and recommended that I treat the disorder with a topical steroid and antibiotics for three months—but he also admitted that the condition would likely reoccur.

During this same time, I also had a digestion problem. I was bloating after meals and had developed gastric reflux that was so bothersome I needed to sit upright to sleep at night (which in turn meant I felt lethargic during the day). I also had a follow-up bone density test. Over a three-year period I had lost approximately 6 percent bone density in my lumbar spine.

The skin is the largest organ of the body, and because we can see it, any problems it manifests can often serve as a sign that things might be wrong somewhere else. When I considered the fact that my skin, my bones, and my GI tract were all having problems simultaneously, I found it hard to believe that it was the result of three separate, individual conditions, or that treating just the *symptoms* would resolve them. So rather than going the conventional route with medications, even though my diet was already very clean, I decided to put myself on a cleanse-and-elimination diet that removed the most likely food stressors: dairy, gluten, caffeine, sugar, soy, and alcohol. I also started taking hydrochloric acid (HCl) supplements with my meals. Within *one week* the ten months of worsening perioral dermatitis cleared up, and after another two weeks it was completely healed. My new diet, along with the HCl, also stopped my stomach bloating and gastric reflux, and I no longer needed to sit upright to sleep.

Two years later, my bone loss had stabilized; I had sustained no additional decrease in bone density. But why such extensive bone loss in the first place? I believe it was GI-related, in part caused by food sensitivities and primarily caused by hypochlorhydria (insufficient stomach acid). My stomach was not making enough HCl to properly break down protein and to facilitate absorption of calcium at the levels needed for my bones. The usual prescription offered to people who have gastric reflux is a proton pump inhibitor such as Nexium or Prilosec, which inhibits the production of hydrochloric acid in the stomach. So why would taking hydrochloric acid cure my particular brand of stomach bloating and gastric reflux? You will find the answer to that question later in the chapter.

The GI system (see Figure 9.1 on the following page) is intimately connected to bone health. This chapter explains the basics of that system, the symptoms that point to problems in the system, and the steps you can take to improve both your digestion and your bones. We'll begin with an overview of how the digestive system functions when it's working properly.

A Tour of the Digestive System: How Food Gets Turned into Healthy Bone

The digestive process is extremely complex, involving actions of the nervous system, hormones, digestive juices, and several organs. To get a better idea of why healthy digestion is so important to our bones, let's take a look at the major players that digest the foods we eat into particles so small that the cells of our bones can absorb them. The

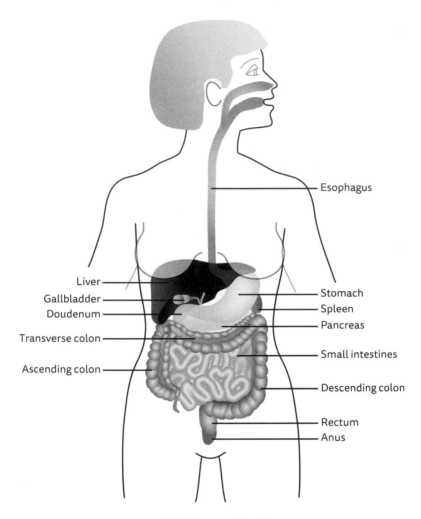

FIGURE 9.1. The human digestive system

digestive process can be broken into four phases: cephalic (involving the brain), oral (involving the mouth), gastric (involving the stomach), and intestinal (involving the small and large intestines). Let's see what happens to food as it goes through these phases, and let's also assume that the food ingested is in fact nutritious—that it has not been overly processed, which would result in a product almost devoid of nutrition.

First we start with the brain.

Cephalic (Brain) Phase

As this term suggests, digestion begins before food is even ingested. The thought or smell of food starts the process in the brain, where neurons signal various glands and the stomach to begin secreting hormones, HCl, and enzymes in anticipation of the food that's on its way.

What are enzymes? They are biological catalysts. They attach to a specific site on a substance in order to speed up a chemical reaction such as digestion. Most, but not all, enzyme names end with the suffix -*ase*.

Oral Phase

The oral phase starts when we begin to chew (masticate) our food, breaking down larger pieces into smaller ones. Chewing and taste tell the salivary glands to secrete saliva, which not only moistens the food but also releases a bicarbonate buffer (to neutralize acidic foods) and the digestive enzyme amylase (to begin digesting starch).

Like the sight or thought of food, the taste of food and the sensation of food in the mouth stimulate the release of hormones, enzymes, and other digestive fluids in the stomach. Once the food leaves the mouth it travels down the esophagus to the stomach, where it enters the gastric phase of digestion. Food that has left the mouth to continue on the digestive process is referred to as a bolus.

Gastric Phase

When the bolus reaches the stomach it triggers the release of the hormone gastrin, which in turn both stimulates and regulates the release of hydrochloric acid (HCl). HCl is a powerful digestive tool; it breaks down large food particles into smaller ones and also destroys undesirable bacteria that may have entered with the food or from some other source. It also converts pepsinogen, an enzyme precursor released by the stomach, into the active enzyme pepsin, which specifically targets proteins, breaking them down further.

The stomach can take two to four hours to empty following a meal. The length of time a substance remains in the stomach depends on the substance. Carbohydrates and liquids exit first, followed by protein, fat, and fibrous foods. (Carbohydrate, protein, and fat are collectively known as macronutrients.) Once the bolus has reached the stage where it is a thick, semifluid mass of partially digested food—referred to as chyme—it passes from the stomach into the first section of the small intestine, the duodenum.

Intestinal Phase

The intestines have two main parts, the small intestine and the large intestine.

Small Intestine

The small intestine can be fifteen to twenty-three feet long and has three sections: the duodenum, the jejunum, and the ileum. Once the chyme enters the duodenum the hydrochloric acid in which it is saturated triggers the cells of the duodenum to secrete the hormone secretin. Secretin in turn stimulates the pancreas and the gallbladder to release specific enzymes and other fluids that further break down macronutrients.

- *Pancreas:* Important enzymes released by the pancreas include proteases, which break down proteins into amino acids; amylases, which break down carbohydrates (starches) into simple sugars; lipases, which break down lipids (fats) into fatty acids; and nucleases, which break down nucleic acids. The pancreas also secretes bicarbonate, which buffers the acidic chyme. Chyme is bathed in HCl in the stomach as a normal part of the digestive process, but if too much acid enters the duodenum over a long period of time, an ulcer can develop. Ulcers occur most often in the duodenum. The pancreas is also the source of the very important hormone insulin, which is central to enabling the body's cells to process carbohydrates and fat.

- *Gallbladder:* The gallbladder stores and later releases bile, a bitter-tasting, greenish fluid that's produced in the liver. Bile is mostly water with bile salts and a small amount of mucus and pigment. Fat stimulates the gallbladder's release of bile into the duodenum, and the bile then emulsifies (breaks up) the fat for easy absorption into the bloodstream.

Interestingly, the intestinal wall itself also secretes enzymes and digestive aids. One of the most important enzymes secreted by the intestinal wall is lactase, which breaks down lactose, a sugar in milk.

After passing the ducts that connect the gallbladder and pancreas to the duodenum, the chyme continues on its journey by means of wave-like muscle contractions called peristalsis. Aiding the chyme's movement are finger-like projections, or villi, that jut out of the lining of the small intestine. In addition to helping the chyme move through the small intestine, the villi have another very significant role: Their shape increases the surface area through which nutrients are absorbed by a whopping 600 percent.

The intestines absorb the nutrients from food by way of specialized receptors that allow only certain nutrients to pass. For example, calcium and magnesium are absorbed in the duodenum, vitamin C and sugars are absorbed in the jejunum, and vitamin B-12, proteins, and fats are absorbed in the ileum (see Figure 9.2 on the following page).

Bacteria in the Gut

Both the small and large intestines are teeming with healthy bacteria whose main role is to assist in the breakdown of undigested carbohydrates. It is essential to keep the "good" bacteria that aid digestion in balance if the digestive tract is to remain healthy and nutrients are to be absorbed properly. For example, the absorption of B-12 is aided by healthy gut flora. Many older adults are deficient in this vitamin, and studies have shown that B-12 deficiency is one of the risk factors associated with bone loss. In Chapter 10 we will discuss how to keep these gut critters in balance to make sure you harbor enough of the good guys.

Large Intestine

Like the small intestine, the large intestine, or colon, also has three segments: the ascending colon, the transverse colon, and the descending colon. The entire large intestine is approximately five to seven feet long and about three inches wide. With its resident bacterial population, it is more than just a waste-storage facility; in fact, the colon has four major functions:

1. reabsorption of water and mineral ions (e.g., sodium, chloride)

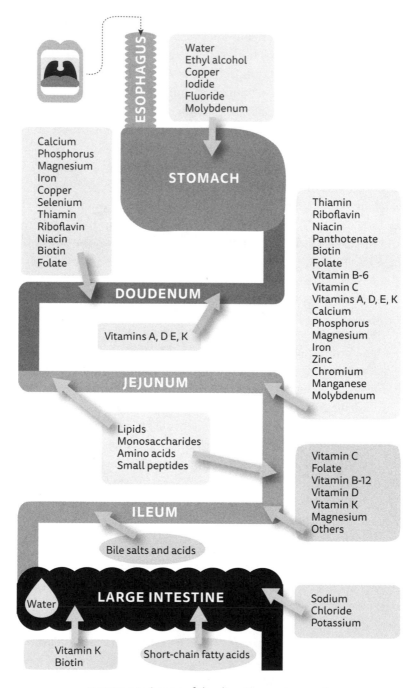

FIGURE 9.2. A map of the digestive system and
corresponding nutrient absorption sites

2. maintenance of a population of over five hundred species of bacteria

3. fermentation of indigestible materials

4. temporary storage of feces

The bacteria living in the colon play a central role in its contribution to the digestive process. Interestingly, vitamin K-2 is made from bacteria in the large intestine and is also absorbed in the large intestine.

Once the digestive process is complete, the remaining material is stored in the descending colon until we defecate, at which point what is evacuated is a fairly large stool that is soft yet "held together." Because it was stored in the colon, which consists of many *S* shaped curves, the stool might have a slight *S* curve.

Remember, as we started this abridged tour of the digestive tract, we assumed that everything in the system was in top-notch condition. What happens when the digestive system is not in good shape? The signs and symptoms of GI problems are discussed in the following section, followed by a look at some of the most common causes of these problems.

How Do You Know If You Have a Digestive Problem?

How do you know if your digestive system is not working as it should? The symptoms to watch for—for example, flatulence, diarrhea, constipation, and heartburn—can occur occasionally in people with perfectly healthy digestion. But they should be infrequent issues, not constant burdens. In fact, it is extremely common for women to experience loose stools or constipation around their menstrual cycle or during pregnancy as a result of hormonal changes. As is the case with most bodily systems, the occasional irregularity in the GI system doesn't indicate a chronic issue, just as an occasional headache doesn't signify a brain tumor. But symptoms such as those listed below that occur daily or even weekly are signs that something is impacting the digestive tract—something that, over time, could lead to problems throughout the entire body.

Some of the most common signs and symptoms of gastrointestinal problems include:

o excessive gas, bloating, burping, or flatulence

o heartburn or GERD

o food sensitivities

o stomach cramps or nausea

o abnormal stools

o abnormal bowel habits (e.g., constipation, diarrhea, taking a long time to void the bowels)

o itching or burning of the rectum

Furthermore, other chronic symptoms that most people don't think of as GI-related can also indicate a problem in the GI system, for example:

o skin irritations, rashes, eczema

o headaches

o fatigue

o anxiety or depression

o joint or muscle pain

o unexplained weight gain or weight loss

Please note that I am not saying these additional "vague" symptoms are *necessarily* GI-related—but they might be, depending on their cause. Weight gain, for example, can be caused by insufficient intake or absorption of the B vitamins, iron, magnesium, and other nutrients needed to help the body burn calories. Bottom line: If your body is not getting the nutrients it needs, you may experience a wide range of problems—and not just those we typically think of as tied to the digestive tract.

Where to Look First:
Taking the Taboo Out of Poo

The head bone's connected to the neck bone, the neck bone's connected to the backbone—and they're all connected to the gut. In my practice, one of the first things I assess when I see a patient who presents with bone loss is their digestive health. Before their initial visit, along with completing a nine-page questionnaire, my new patients are tasked with keeping a seven-day diet and symptom journal, which gives me an idea of their food choices, nutrient intake, and digestive health. (You can access this log on my website, through the Forms link.) During a patient's first appointment, I candidly discuss their GI symptoms, and some of the most important questions I ask concern their bowel movements. Granted, the topic is not one most people want to discuss, but knowing about someone's stools gives me a lot of information about how their digestive tract may or may not be working.

Everyone has abnormal bowel movements from time to time due to illness or as a reaction to a food substance (or something else) that has been ingested. However, if you have abnormal bowel movements on a regular basis, it may be a significant sign that something is not right with your body. Color, odor, texture, and consistency are all aspects of a person's stool that can provide clues about whether or not the GI tract is working as it should. Following is a brief overview of what to look for when it comes to bowel movements.

Color

Color tells us a lot about when stools are abnormal. The color of a healthy stool is brownish, but a white or very pale-colored stool, for example, can indicate that the gallbladder is not releasing enough bile (bile has a greenish color, which darkens the stool). Red streaks, red spots, or other reddish areas in the stool may indicate the presence of blood from either the descending colon or the rectum. Blood that has travelled from the stomach or intestines may produce dark or blackish stools. The most common cause of red blood in stools is a bleeding hemorrhoid, but blood in the stool can also be an early warning sign of cancer, so don't ignore it. Red beets can produce red stool (and urine), and Pepto-Bismol can cause very dark stool.

Constipation

Everyone has experienced constipation from time to time; it is one of the conditions with which my patients most often present. Some of the symptoms include abdominal pain, gas, and bloating, but constipation can also cause fatigue and even permanent damage to the colon. Although occasional constipation is nothing to worry about, pain with bowel movements or straining on a regular basis is not normal; a bowel movement should be effortless. Following are some of the main causes of constipation:

- ◦ dehydration
- ◦ insufficient magnesium intake
- ◦ a low-fiber diet
- ◦ diverticulosis (out-pocketing in the large intestine)
- ◦ hemorrhoids
- ◦ irritable bowel syndrome (IBS)
- ◦ excessive intake of protein and/or dairy products
- ◦ hypochlorhydria (low production of hydrochloric acid in the stomach)
- ◦ insufficient physical activity
- ◦ pelvic floor dysfunction (caused when the muscles that are used to move the bowels aren't properly coordinated)
- ◦ certain hormonal disturbances, for example, hypothyroidism
- ◦ certain medications, for example, those that contain codeine (always read drug labels for possible side effects)

For many people, constipation can be easily fixed with dietary and lifestyle changes that include whole foods, more exercise, more water, fiber-rich foods, and enough magnesium in the diet to balance calcium. (You'll learn how to balance these two minerals in Chapter 10.)

Loose Stools

Diarrhea, or loose stools, can be caused by digestive disorders, infections, or dietary intake of certain foods or food additives. Whereas everyone experiences transient episodes of loose stools from time to time, chronic diarrhea means that you may not be absorbing the nutrients you need, which in turn can lead to significant problems—for example, bone loss. Some of the main causes of chronic diarrhea include:

o high intake of sugar alcohols, found in diet drinks and diet foods (if you're someone who reads food labels, watch for ingredients such as xylitol, sorbitol, mannitol, lactitol, isomalt, maltitol, or hydrogenated starch hydrolysates)

o poor diet choices or overindulgence in certain foods, especially sugar and greasy junk foods such as potato chips

o candida overgrowth (candida is a yeast that lives in the intestines; see below for more information)

o certain medications, including antibiotics, antidepressants such as Zoloft and Prozac, and corticosteroids (e.g., prednisone)

o certain food intolerances (for example, lactose intolerance or celiac disease)

o pancreatic insufficiency (which leads to low output of digestive enzymes)

o gallbladder impairment (which leads to low output of the gallbladder's digestive juices)

o irritable bowel syndrome (IBS)

o leaky gut syndrome

o autoimmune diseases of the intestines, for example, Crohn's disease, ulcerative colitis, or celiac disease

o food poisoning

o infections

Mucus

Whitish mucus in the stool may be a sign of an intestinal disease. Small amounts of mucus in the stool are normal, but irritable bowel syndrome, celiac disease, diverticulitis, ulcerative colitis, bacterial infections, and Crohn's disease may lead to amounts that are greater than normal.

Fatty Stool

Steatorrhea, or the presence of excessive fat in the stools, is one of the main signs of malabsorption conditions such as gluten intolerance (described in more detail later in the chapter). Fatty stools are often oily and foul smelling; they may float or stick to the side of the bowl, making it difficult to flush them away.

○○◯○○

The Bristol Stool Chart is another tool that can help you identify whether your stools are normal. The chart classifies human stool in terms of seven categories, using both illustrations and written descriptions to describe each stool form. The Bristol stool types are described in Table 9.1 below, and you can also find the chart on my website, www.LaniSimpson.com.

Table 9.1. The Bristol Stool Types

Type	Description	Analysis
Type 1	Separate, hard lumps, like nuts. Hard to pass, indicating constipation.	Abnormal
Type 2	Sausage-shaped and lumpy. Hard to pass, indicating constipation.	Abnormal
Type 3	Sausage-shaped with cracks on the surface, leaning toward constipation.	Abnormal
Type 4	Sausage-shaped or snake-shaped, smooth, and soft. May have a curve. Easy to pass.	Normal
Type 5	Soft blobs with clear-cut edges.	A normal variant
Type 6	Fluffy pieces with ragged edges, mushy, leaning toward diarrhea.	Borderline abnormal
Type 7	Watery, no solid pieces.	Abnormal

The Bristol stool chart is a useful tool; however, it does not include important symptoms such as color or odor, and there is some disagreement as to the normality or abnormality of some of the types. For example, some experts view type 3 as normal. In my opinion, and that of other health-care practitioners, this type is not normal but rather indicates a mild form of constipation.

Bowel movements should be effortless, and they should occur at least once a day. Some medical references state that constipation is defined by a failure to defecate within a three-day period. I strongly disagree with this assessment. Though failure to defecate once each day may be the norm in a society that eats a typical American diet, it indicates suboptimal functioning. In fact, a diet that is high in fiber usually produces more than one healthy bowel movement each day.

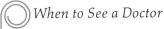 *When to See a Doctor*

See your primary care provider if you have a significant change in bowel movements. Pencil-thin stool or blood in the stool is another reason to see a doctor. Pencil-thin stools can be a sign of bowel obstruction, internal bleeding can cause black or very dark stool, and red blood in the stool can be caused by hemorrhoids or bleeding from the colon. Chronic GI problems cannot be cured with over-the-counter drugs, which treat only the symptoms. If you have chronic GI problems, have them assessed and diagnosed.

What Causes GI Problems?

Chronic or acute problems in the gut can be the result of chemical exposure, hormonal or microbial imbalances, or structural problems, and can occur at any point along the digestive tract. This section provides a brief overview of some of the most common causes of GI dysfunction.

Food Intolerances, Sensitivities, and Allergies

There is a lot of confusion about what constitutes a food intolerance, food allergy, or food sensitivity and about how each of them can impact a person's ability to digest food and absorb nutrients. The nutrient value of one's diet is *very* important; things like vitamin or mineral deficiencies can cause serious issues, as can an overabundance of proteins and carbohydrates or a shortage of fiber. I discuss the importance of diet and nutrition in more detail in the next chapter, but for now, know that even if you are eating foods that normally are considered healthy, if you have a food intolerance, food sensitivity, or food allergy, it may be that those "healthy" foods are the cause of your GI symptoms.

Although food allergies, food intolerances, and food sensitivities are separate conditions, the terms are often misapplied, so let me explain the differences.

Food intolerances: The term "food intolerance" refers to an adverse reaction either to a specific food or to certain ingredients or compounds found in the food. As you'll see below, food intolerances are different from allergies. Food intolerances occur for several different reasons; some are caused by defects in the digestive process—for example, when the body lacks an enzyme needed to digest the "problem" food. Food intolerances can result in multiple GI symptoms. A food-intolerant person feels best when they avoid the foods that trigger a reaction, but most of the reactions aren't caused by the immune system and are not life threatening.

One food intolerance many people develop as they grow older is lactose intolerance. Lactose is a sugar contained in milk products; it is broken down in the body by the enzyme lactase. Lactose intolerance arises from the body's inability to produce lactase, which is known to dwindle after age forty. Lactose intolerance is common in much of the world's population, most significantly among African Americans, Latinos, Asians, and Native Americans. Symptoms of lactose intolerance can include bloating after eating, gurgling sounds in the lower abdomen, and diarrhea. Those who have difficulty digesting most dairy products may be able to eat yogurt that is made with active bacterial cultures, which produce lactase; traditional yogurt also has a relatively low lactose content.

Another common food intolerance is gluten intolerance, also known as celiac disease (CD). CD is an inherited autoimmune disease (with environmental components) that can manifest as an extreme intolerance to gluten, a protein found in wheat, barley, rye, and spelt. Gluten may also be present on other grains, especially oats, that have been harvested or processed using the same equipment that was used to process gluten-containing grains. CD, a lifelong condition, if left untreated, leads to destruction of the villi that line the small intestine, which in turn causes malabsorption and, ultimately, bone loss. Some of the signs of CD include weight loss and steatorrhea. Patients with osteoporosis should always be evaluated for celiac disease. People with CD must avoid gluten. CD can be diagnosed with certain blood tests (see Chapter 5 for information about testing), although these tests are not completely reliable. A biopsy of the small intestine can also be used diagnose CD. Eliminating all gluten sources from the diet is also diagnostic.

Food sensitivities (FS): The body's reaction to food sensitivities tends to be less severe than its reaction to food intolerances or allergies, and FS may or may not result in GI symptoms. FS can emerge when certain foods are eaten in excess, particularly when they are eaten regularly over long periods; for that reason, food sensitivities tend to occur with the foods we crave and eat frequently. There are a variety of symptoms associated with food sensitivities, including:

- GI symptoms, for example, irritable bowel syndrome (IBS), constipation, diarrhea, or nausea
- bloating, gas, extreme abdominal discomfort
- weight gain or unexplained weight loss
- skin problems such as rashes, hives, and eczema
- respiratory problems such as sinusitis, asthma, sore throat, or persistent cough
- fungal infections such as thrush, jock itch, or ringworm

Less is known about food sensitivities that don't result in GI problems. Since their effects are often gradual rather than immediate and may be far removed from the digestive arena, they can be hard to diagnose without lab testing and/or elimination diets. Still, food sensitivities are quite common, and they can intensify over time, causing chronic health problems. In extreme cases, they may even trigger asthma attacks. The cure for most food sensitivities is to remove the offending food from the diet for three months to a year. After the food has been removed for a sufficient period of time, it can often be tolerated if eaten only occasionally.

Many of my patients are surprised to find out they have a food sensitivity: "But I've been eating that food my whole life!" It is common to develop sensitivities to certain foods as we age. FS can also be triggered during times of stress or illness, or any time the immune system is compromised.

Food allergies: A true allergy always results in a positive blood test for immunoglobulin E (IgE). Food allergies are much less common than food intolerances and food sensitivities, occurring in approximately 5 percent of the population. They are considered to be a fixed condition, meaning that the allergic reaction occurs every time the food is eaten. Some of the symptoms of food allergies include swelling in the mouth, asthma, and even anaphylactic shock, which could result in death. Food allergies can be life-threatening.

As shown above, food allergies, food intolerances, and food sensitivities are different entities. If you're having a reaction to a particular food substance, it is important for you to find out which condition is causing the reaction if you are to manage your symptoms effectively. To do this you'll need to work with a doctor who understands how to test for these different conditions. Allergists, for example, often rely on skin tests to identify allergens, but a skin test typically does not pinpoint food sensitivities.

Some of the tests that can help to identify the cause of a food reaction include:

o hydrogen breath testing for lactose intolerance and fructose malabsorption

o elimination diets (see below)

o testing for immunoglobulin G- (IgG) and immunoglobulin E- (IgE) mediated immune responses to specific foods

o stool testing for yeast and/or bacterial overgrowth

See Resources for reliable testing labs.

Issues with Acid

Above, we saw how GI problems can occur simply as a result of the body's responses to particular foods. In the rest of the section, the conditions we address are presented as problems of the digestive tract itself. Notice, however, that this distinction is not as clear-cut as it may seem. As described above, for example, one reason why we may be unable to tolerate a food substance is because our digestive system lacks the enzyme(s) needed to properly digest it. And as you'll see below, some GI conditions—for example, excessive permeability of the intestinal wall—can be caused by poor diet. So in some cases, digestive tract dysfunction can be seen as a response to certain foods.

We begin our discussion with an overview of hyperchlorhydria (excess stomach acid) and hypochlorhydria (low stomach acid).

GERD (gastroesophageal reflux disease): GERD is most commonly caused by chronic acid reflux, or the regular, frequent regurgitation of stomach acid or bile into the esophagus (food pipe). The primary symptom of GERD is heartburn, or a burning sensation in the upper stomach region. But GERD can also be silent; that is, not everyone experiences burning, although they may have other symptoms. Hoarseness, sinus infections, and even asthma can be caused by GERD. Chronic acid reflux can erode the cells in the lower esophagus, leading to Barrett's esophagus, a condition characterized by the presence of precancerous cells. If you do experience burning and if you have GERD, some dietary changes, which you will learn about in Chapter 10, may be all you need to resolve the condition.

Hypochlorhydria: "Tum, Tum-Tum-Tum, Tums!" Those of you who remember this jingle know that Tums is an antacid that's designed to stop heartburn. But wait—remember my experience with gastric reflux, which I shared at the beginning of this chapter? Even though doctors often treat heartburn or GERD with antacids, which are designed to neutralize stomach acidity, gastric reflux can also be caused by *insufficient* stomach acid (hypochlorhydria). Food can remain in the stomach for longer periods when acid levels are too low, possibly leading to fermentation of the food. This may or may not cause burning sensations in the abdomen.

It is common for stomach acid (HCl) levels to decrease with age, so in some cases, especially if a person suffers from chronic bloating right after eating, the issue may be a lack of enough stomach acid to properly digest food. Antacids, then, would only make the symptoms worse. Not only that, they would contribute to additional GI problems as well. For example, as we saw earlier, one of HCl's main roles is to break down food into smaller particles. If, due to low HCl levels, the body's ability to break food down is compromised, food will pass through the body in a relatively undigested state, leaving the person deprived of the nutrients the food would have provided. Testing for hypochlorhydria (sometimes called "hypochloridia") is simple and inexpensive, requiring only experimentation with HCl supplements to determine their impact on symptoms. However, because too much HCl in the system is also a serious problem, I strongly suggest that you do not engage in testing unless you're working with a health professional who is familiar with GI health. (*Note:* Chronic use of ibuprofen, aspirin, and some other medications damage [thin] the stomach lining, making it more susceptible to injury from even normal HCl levels.)

H. pylori: A common stomach bacterium that was discovered in 1982, *H. pylori* thrives when stomach acid levels are low. *H. pylori* has been found to be the main cause of most stomach ulcers and other symptoms of acute infection, including gastritis, heartburn, and nausea and discomfort after eating. Infection is easy to test for through the blood, stool, and urine, and even via a breath test. Anyone who suspects an ulcer should always see a medical professional. An adequate level of HCl is one of the body's first defenses against this bacterium.

"Dropping Acid" to Resolve Reflux: John's Story
Seventy-year-old John came to me with a history of osteoporosis as well as chronic GI symptoms he'd been battling for over ten years. His GI symptoms included constipation, bloating, belching, and occasional gastric reflux, and he had been on proton pump inhibitors (PPIs) for five years in an attempt to treat the problems.

PPIs (for example, Nexium and Prilosec) are medications that stop the body from producing stomach acid. Lowering a patient's stomach acid levels can be useful if he or she has chronic acid reflux (GERD), because prolonged exposure to acid can result in permanent, severe damage to the esophagus. But John said that his GI symptoms had never included any burning sensations. Moreover, he wasn't sure if his medications were actually helping; he reported that at one point he stopped taking them and felt fewer symptoms without them. John went back on the meds when his doctor warned that gastric reflux could damage his esophagus. John's doctor had never evaluated his diet or other factors to see if it was possible to address his symptoms without medication.

At my prompting, John began keeping a detailed log of his diet and symptoms. We learned that whereas his reflux was only occasional, significant bloating and belching happened nightly, after he ate large, protein-rich dinners. (John typically ate a small breakfast of toast, milk, and coffee. He also skipped lunch at times, and then consumed a very large amount of food at dinner to compensate for having eaten so little during the day.)

My first step was to introduce a change in John's eating schedule, managing his food intake to include three smaller meals and two healthy snacks each day. We implemented a whole-food diet that eliminated most of the processed foods he had been eating, and also added a small-dose supplement of hydrochloric acid to his main meals.

Within one month, John's symptoms had improved dramatically. I suggested that he tell his doctor about the work he and I were doing. He did so, and his doctor began to wean him from the PPI he'd been taking. John continued to use HCl in fairly high doses, and, of course, his dietary changes also played an important role in his improvement. One month later, John reported that he was symptom free and that he had more energy than he remembered ever having.

Other Common GI Conditions

Hypochlorhydria, *H. pylori*, GERD... These conditions can serve as a reminder of just how important it is that the gastric (stomach) phase of digestion functions as it should. In particular, if we don't have enough stomach acid, or if we have a condition that allows for acid to move to parts of the body where it shouldn't be, any of several painful GI conditions can follow. Furthermore, low stomach acid keeps the body from breaking down food into nutrients that can be absorbed. Other common conditions that can keep the body from accessing the nutrients in food are inflammatory bowel disease, leaky gut syndrome, irritable bowel syndrome, gastritis, and flora imbalances. These conditions are described below.

Inflammatory bowel disease (IBD): The term "inflammatory bowel disease" does not refer to a single condition but instead is considered a category of inflammatory diseases of the intestines. The most common types of IBD are Crohn's disease and ulcerative colitis. Symptoms of IBD include those that are common to GI problems—for example, diarrhea, cramping, vomiting, abdominal pain—as well as anemia. IBD is an autoimmune disease that develops as a result of both genetic and environmental factors.

Irritable bowel syndrome (IBS): IBS, or spastic colon, can be caused by any number of irritations. Symptoms include bloating, abdominal pain, diarrhea, and constipation. IBS is not an inflammatory condition and in my experience will often clear up once the diet is cleaned up. Eating a bone-healthy diet such as the one described in Chapter 10 will go a long way to healing the condition in most people.

Leaky gut syndrome (LG): Leaky gut, or increased intestinal permeability, is recognized in both conventional and alternative medicine. It can be caused by toxins, parasites, poor diet, infections, or intestinal diseases such as celiac or Crohn's disease. A leaky gut allows substances such as toxins, microbes, undigested food, waste, or larger-than-normal macromolecules to leak through an abnormally permeable gut wall. These out-of-place substances can either affect the body directly (e.g., as in the case of toxins or waste) or initiate an autoimmune reaction. Long-term intestinal permeability may also result in malabsorption of nutrients, although there is disagreement as to whether other health conditions are caused or merely exacerbated by LG.

Gastritis: Gastritis, or inflammation of the stomach lining, can be chronic or acute. Many conditions can lead to chronic gastritis, including *H. pylori* infection, excessive alcohol use, stress, food sensitivities, or the short- or long-term use of certain medications, such as aspirin or ibuprofen—or the medications used to treat osteoporosis. Oral bisphosphonates have been known to cause significant damage to the stomach and/or the esophagus in susceptible individuals.

Flora imbalances: Another common cause of GI problems is the overgrowth of flora in the intestines. Though our bodies need the "good" flora that help us with digestion, any microbial imbalance can hinder nutrient absorption. A type of fungus we often hear about when it comes to microbial overgrowth is the candida yeast. The term "candida" refers to a category of fungi; *Candida albicans* is one of several such yeasts that live in the intestines. *Candida albicans* is known to cause infections in both humans and animals, although for most of us it poses no adverse effects. However, when factors such as long-term antibiotic use, high carbohydrate consumption, or immune-compromising conditions cause a decline in the intestinal flora that keep this yeast in check, it can run rampant. Overabundant intestinal flora steal nutrients from the intestines to use for their own growth, leading to symptoms such as bloating, fatigue, mental cloudiness, and sugar cravings, among others.

"I've been told I have a malabsorption condition. What does that mean?"

Not surprisingly, the term "malabsorption" refers to a dysfunction in the absorption of nutrients. If you've been told you have a malabsorption condition, it means that even if the food you're eating is perfectly balanced and highly nutritious, your body is not getting the nutrients it needs from the food.

Diarrhea and steatorrhea are two of the most common symptoms of malabsorption, but its causes are many. They include some of the conditions discussed in this chapter, for example, celiac disease, lactose intolerance, and IBD. Other causes are listed below, but please note that this list is not all-inclusive:

- hyperthyroidism or hypothyroidism
- bacterial overgrowth or parasites
- pancreatic insufficiencies
- enzyme deficiencies
- fructose malabsorption
- malnutrition

(cont'd.)

- surgical changes; for example, removal of part of the intestines or stomach

- infective agents; for example, HIV or parasites

Over time, malabsorption conditions can have serious consequences for your health, including the health of your bones. As I've emphasized throughout this chapter, in order for your bones to be healthy they must receive all of the bone-building nutrients they require. Malabsorption conditions in younger people impair their ability to build bone, and in older people decrease bone quality or cause bone loss. If you or your doctor suspect that you have a malabsorption condition, it will be important to test for the specific underlying causes that may have led to the problem. One test that's especially useful in this regard is the stool test, which can identify infectious agents and disease processes that lead to malabsorption.

Treating the Body Rather Than the Symptoms: A Blueprint for Healthy Digestion

So far in this chapter we've discussed some of the main GI-related problems that can keep a person from getting the nutrients they need to maintain healthy bones. What should you do if you have one (or more) of these conditions? Unfortunately, the solution isn't as simple as taking a pill to make the disorder disappear. After all, you didn't get here overnight; for many folks, GI conditions are the result of lifestyle and eating patterns whose long-term effects take years and sometimes even decades to develop. It makes sense, then, that resolving such conditions is also a process requiring substantive dietary and lifestyle changes. The healing process can take time. This section describes some of the key eating habits that can begin to correct the health of your digestive tract, thus improving your digestion and absorption.

Because the failure to maintain a balanced, nutritious diet can lead to numerous GI-related symptoms, it can be difficult to pinpoint the exact cause of a digestive problem, especially if one's diet is high in processed carbohydrates, sugar, caffeine, or alcohol. Along the same lines, most people can improve their symptoms by switching to a whole-foods diet that includes few or no processed foods, foods that are low in salt and sugar, and plenty of water—though this is not always the case. Some GI problems are congenital, for example, and chronic nutritional deficits can result in permanent problems. Although a relatively small percentage of individuals may be unable to reduce their symptoms by changing what they eat, it is absolutely the case that healthy digestion begins with putting the right nutrients into the body.

Eat Real Food

Michael Pollan writes in his book *The Omnivore's Dilemma,* "Eat food. Not too much. Mostly plants." These words of advice can serve as a succinct guide for eating that truly supports digestion. With regard to "food," Pollan is referring to the real stuff, the groceries found in the outer aisles of the store, the foods that can go bad and are made up of ingredients you can see. We've spoken about how gluten, dairy, and some complex carbohydrates can lead to certain GI conditions; some individuals must entirely steer clear of these substances. But even for those of us without chronic GI conditions there are some foods that should be consumed only occasionally—if not avoided altogether. Sugar and processed carbohydrates top this list, and caffeine and alcohol should also be kept to a minimum. I discuss food and nutrition in much more detail in Chapter 10; for now just keep in mind that eating "real" foods is a critical component to keeping your digestive system on track.

Don't Overdo It

We've all heard, and most of us believe, that overeating can have a negative impact on our health. This is true in a general sense; for example, excess weight gained through chronic overeating places undue stress on the heart. Overeating also exacerbates the problems that result when what we're overeating is junk food, or even too much of a certain type of "nourishing" food, such as meat or bread. When I talk with my patients about habits that can improve digestion, I like to point to the example set by the Okinawan people, who have the longest life expectancy on earth. Okinawan elders have a simple saying that describes their eating philosophy: *Hara hachi bu.* Translated, this means: "Eat until you are eight parts full." Okinawans do not stuff themselves at meals; instead, they eat several small meals per day. Supplement companies market coral calcium and related nutrients with the promise that if we just take their products we'll enjoy a life span to rival to that of the Okinawans, who often live to be one hundred. Rather than focusing on a single substance, however, I think it's a great idea to emulate the *lifestyle* habits of such individuals.

Of course, the Okinawan approach to eating includes other healthy habits that no doubt also contribute to their long lifespan. Their diet is rich in fermented foods, vegetables, fruits, fish, soy, and green tea. Okinawans also get plenty of exercise, and their elders are respected rather than forgotten, which undoubtedly adds to the quality of their lives and probably to their lifespan as well.

Emphasize Plant Foods

So far this chapter has devoted a fair amount of attention to the importance of *avoiding* certain foods. So what do you eat instead? It should come as no surprise that for optimum GI health, half if not more of your caloric intake should come from primarily vegetables and some fruits. Fruits and vegetables are the main sources of many of the vitamins and minerals our bodies need (you will read more about this in Chapter 10); they help reduce risk for heart disease, osteoporosis, and diabetes; they provide protection against certain cancers; those that are rich in potassium may lower blood pressure and may protect against kidney stones and bone loss; and the dietary fiber found in plants is absolutely essential to proper GI function. In the words of David Katz, MD, director of the Yale Prevention Research Center, "[P]lants—vegetables, fruits, nuts, seeds, beans, lentils, whole grains...are decisively associated with better health."

One of the principal diet trends is the raw food diet. Proponents of this diet maintain that cooking food to temperatures over 115 degrees Fahrenheit destroys plant enzymes that could be healthy for us. There is some controversy regarding how beneficial plant enzymes are for the human body. That said, I do think that eating raw foods is a healthy practice.

Practice Mindful Eating

In today's world many of us tend to rush just about everything, but for optimal digestion meals should be savored. One of the practices that helped me to eat more slowly is what's known as "mindful eating meditation." Being more mindful while eating—taking the time to practice intentional, focused awareness on the simple process of eating—helps us to observe and experience more fully whether and how we nourish ourselves. I believe that it's not really possible to make unhealthy food choices on a regular basis if we are truly "present" when we choose our foods.

I encourage you to practice mindful eating meditation with one meal or one snack each day. Have at least one meal a day without any distractions. That means no radio, TV, reading, or conversation. Eat in silence. Begin by setting up a disruption-free environment. Notice what you are choosing to eat, and notice the portions you put on your plate. Next:

- Take a few deep breaths before beginning to eat.
- When you start to eat, be aware of how the food feels in the mouth, fully chewing each bite before swallowing.
- Notice how the food tastes. Really paying attention to the taste of food often shows us that the flavor is more complex than we've realized.
- Notice when you are approximately 80 percent full, and stop eating. If you decide to continue eating, notice what it feels like to eat more.

Once you have finished eating, notice how your stomach feels. Do you feel full? Does your stomach feel comfortable or uncomfortable? Did the meal satisfy you? Finally, did you make healthy choices at this meal? If not, are you judging yourself for it? What are you telling yourself about the choices you made?

Whether or not you wish your meal had been more nutritious, your eating meditation has much value. Intentional, complete awareness of our food intake can help us to eat healthy food, and cultivating mindfulness of "bad" choices can eventually place limits on such behaviors or stop them altogether.

Therapies That May Aid Digestion

So you have a gastrointestinal problem, and you've taken the first step toward solving that problem: You are now eating the right foods in the right amounts. This step is very important, and I commend you for taking it. But what if you find that you're still having symptoms? Depending on the severity and chronicity of your problem, you may need additional support. Below is a brief description of some of the GI-related tools I recommend to my patients—tools that can help your gut become your ally in your quest for better bone health.

Some of these remedies—for example, an elimination diet or enzyme supplements—are fine to try on your own. On the other hand, it's also very important that your GI problems be accurately diagnosed. Not only do you want to be able to give your body the best treatment for your condition, but, even more important, the wrong treatment can actually make your condition worse. Consider the Tums example from earlier in the chapter. If you have gastric reflux due to insufficient gastric acid (hypochlorhydria), taking Tums or a proton pump inhibitor such as Zantac can aggravate the disorder. Along the same lines, be careful taking HCl supplements. HCl can cause painful burning sensations in the abdominal area and elsewhere, so, as stated, it's a good idea to use this treatment only when you're working with a health care professional who has a solid understanding of digestion and digestive health.

Elimination Diet

As mentioned earlier there are different ways to test for food intolerances, allergies, and sensitivities, including blood, stool, and skin-prick testing. Generally speaking, blood and stool testing are more accurate (see Resources for labs that offer testing); however, an elimination diet of suspect foods is, in my opinion, the best way to determine whether or not you have reactions to specific foods. An elimination diet involves removing suspect foods or ingredients from your diet because you or your doctor thinks they may be the cause of your symptoms. To test, the "problem" foods are eliminated for a period of time in an effort to see if symptoms are alleviated. Some of the more common foods that can cause allergies or sensitivities include: dairy, gluten, eggs, nuts, corn, grains, soy and other legumes, citrus fruits, and nightshade vegetables (tomatoes, peppers, eggplant, potatoes). Caffeine, alcohol, and sugar are also typically eliminated to make sure these are not masking, causing, or contributing to the symptoms you are experiencing.

The amount of time needed to see if your symptoms are alleviated can be immediate but may take seven days or longer, especially if intestinal damage has occurred. After you have eliminated the foods you suspect may be contributing to your symptoms, add the foods back to your diet one at a time, waiting at least one week before reintroducing another food. As you add foods, notice whether symptoms reoccur. If they do—for example, if you experience stomach bloating after reintroducing dairy—you now know that you might have a problem digesting dairy products.

How long must you eliminate suspect foods before you see results? It varies. If you have lactose intolerance, the symptoms will clear up as soon as you stop eating foods that contain dairy. By contrast, if you have celiac disease you may feel better as soon as you stop consuming gluten, or it may take many months to feel symptom free, due to intestinal damage that takes time to heal. If you have a food sensitivity, depending on your symptoms, they, too, may clear up quickly once the offending food is removed. With many food sensitivities you can stop eating the food for six months to a year and then you will be able to resume eating it occasionally. That said, I generally recommend avoiding foods that you are sensitive to. Keep in mind that celiac disease is an autoimmune disease that causes destruction to the small intestine, meaning gluten will need to be removed permanently from the diet. Food sensitivities can also result in intestinal damage over time, especially if the offending foods are eaten in large quantities.

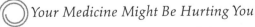

Your Medicine Might Be Hurting You

When addressing GI problems, it's important to be aware of the effects of any medications you are taking. Certain drugs can have a significant negative impact on the digestive system. Antibiotics, for example, can disrupt the body's natural flora, causing an

(cont'd.)

overgrowth of candida. As another example, ibuprofen, aspirin, and oral bisphosphonates (when used frequently) tend to thin the intestines' mucosal lining, impacting the body's ability to absorb nutrients.

But wait! Don't just throw away everything in your medicine cabinet. It is important to work with a professional who can help you decide which medications are necessary (and correctly prescribed) and which are not. And even when this has been determined, there may be a "weaning" period during which you stop taking unwanted medications gradually as opposed to all at once. Certain meds can cause additional problems if you try to quit them cold turkey. If you suspect that your medicine is hurting you, be up front with your practitioner, and ask him or her to work with you to eliminate the unnecessary ones.

Enzyme Supplements

Though the body produces enzymes, supplements can aid in bringing those enzymes to the levels needed to fully digest food. Use of enzyme supplements is often temporary, as the body will produce everything it needs once it is fully nourished with a healthy diet. The enzymes I suggest to my patients depend on the particular conditions they present. I often recommend full-spectrum enzyme supplements that include all of the enzymes needed for digestion. Generally speaking, enzyme supplements are one of those treatments that either will or won't help your digestive problem. They won't harm you, and they may improve things.

Hormone Therapy

Estrogen, progesterone, cortisol, thyroid hormones—these are just a few of the hormones that impact digestion. For this reason, hormonal imbalances and/or age-related decreases in hormone levels can cause or contribute to digestive issues. Bioidentical hormone supplements (discussed in Chapter 8) can sometimes help provide the needed boost to make digestion more efficient; they may also help protect the digestive tract. For example, studies show that estrogen can protect the body from colon cancer in some instances.

Probiotics

If the state of one's intestinal flora is not where it should be, probiotic supplementation can help restore the body's "good bacteria" to optimal levels. Some research suggests that probiotic supplements may help treat a range of GI-related problems, for example, loose stools, constipation, yeast infections, and irritable bowel syndrome. Foods that are rich in natural probiotics include yogurt, fermented cabbage (sauerkraut), kimchi, and other fermented foods. If you're thinking about trying a probiotic supplement, make sure you select one that is refrigerated at the store, and then refrigerate it once at home. It's usually best to take probiotic supplements when your stomach is empty. Be aware that some people feel worse when they add probiotics to their diet, especially those with autoimmune disorders. This being the case, it's a good idea to begin the use of probiotics slowly. In the beginning, you may want to supplement every other day as opposed to every day.

Herbs

Certain herbal supplements can help resolve particular GI-related problems. I often find herbs to be useful in addressing some of my patients' more unique or idiosyncratic symptoms. Below is a list of some of the most common herbs used to improve digestion and/or address GI symptoms:

- o chamomile: an antispasmodic, it relieves stomach cramps, calms the nervous system, and reduces gas and bloating
- o turmeric: stimulates the gallbladder to produce bile, thereby helping with fat digestion
- o lemongrass: calms the digestive system, relieves abdominal pain, and reduces gas and bloating
- o ginger root: improves digestion and relieves nausea and heartburn
- o licorice (deglycerized): reduces the ability of stomach acid to damage the stomach lining by supporting mucosal cells in the stomach lining. Deglycerized licorice, or DGL, will not increase blood pressure

○ fennel seeds: relieve nausea, stomach cramps, indigestion, and bloating, and help to reduce flatulence

○ lemon verbena: improves digestion, relieves stomach and intestinal cramping, reduces gas

○ dandelion root and leaf: improves digestion and acts as a mild laxative

○ yellow dock: stimulates bile production and acts as a mild laxative

○ peppermint: relieves gas; also relieves digestive spasms, reducing pain and discomfort

○ pau d'arco: reduces intestinal yeast overgrowth

As the above list shows, herbs can be used to treat a range of GI problems—but be careful. Herbs are both medicine and food, and you can be allergic to them, just as you can be allergic to anything else you ingest. Make sure you talk to a health-care provider who understands herbs before embarking on a treatment that uses herbs in high doses. Drinking a tea is one thing, but ingesting infusions, which are highly concentrated, can result in adverse effects. It is also important to find out how certain herbs might interact with medications you're taking. For example, some herbs, such as turmeric, act as blood thinners, so it may be unsafe to use them if you are also taking an anticoagulant or antiplatelet medication.

Chiropractic, Acupuncture, Abdominal Massage

For many of my patients, I recommend alternative medical treatments that adjust the body so that the skeleton, muscles, and nerves are aligned in the way they're meant to be. Proper positioning and alignment directly impact the functioning of the various bodily systems. Misalignment in certain areas of the spine, for example, might diminish the performance of the nerves that stimulate digestion. Applying acupuncture or massage to certain anatomic sites can improve functioning and eliminate symptoms. Although treatments such as acupuncture and chiropractic have been disparaged and maligned by many who practice conventional Western medicine, these interventions can and do improve digestion.

○○◯○○

As I have emphasized in this chapter, proper digestion and absorption of nutrients is a key to good health, including bone health. This chapter is certainly not a complete guide to digestive function, and I in no way want to suggest that the reader can self-diagnose with the information presented here. But I do want to give you a clear understanding of just how complex and important digestion is. Sometimes the cure for a digestive condition may be as simple as removing an offending food or taking a supplement. However, if simple remedies do not resolve your condition, I encourage you to see a professional who has an understanding of both gastrointestinal function and nutrition.

Many people think of gastroenterologists as the experts in diagnosis of digestive problems. These specialists can indeed diagnose certain GI problems; however, it has been my experience that many GI doctors do not work with the diet in detail. If the diagnosis is not clearly defined by lab work, rather than looking more closely at nutrition and diet, which can resolve problems at their source, a gastroenterologist may simply offer the patient a medication that addresses only the symptoms.

If you have a digestive problem that you can't solve on your own, you'll benefit immensely from working with a professional who's well versed in nutrition and can guide you in giving your body the nutrients it needs to thrive. If we agree that what matters most to bone health is digestion, digestion, digestion, we must also agree that nutrition, nutrition, nutrition runs a close second—or perhaps even ties. To learn more about how to use food to improve your bone health, keep reading. The next chapter describes how proper nutrition can reduce one's risk for fractures.

 KEY POINTS FROM CHAPTER 9

- Healthy gut bacteria are essential for the health of our body, including our bones.

- Chronic gastrointestinal symptoms are not normal and should be investigated and resolved to the extent possible.

(cont'd.)

- Dehydration is common and is one cause of constipation.

- Hypochlorhydria (low stomach acid) is common in people over age forty and over time may result in bone loss.

- Chronic loose stools can indicate malabsorption, which is a known risk factor for bone loss.

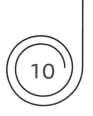

Fight Fractures
with Food

"You are what you eat." Many of us have heard this old adage, and guess what? It's really true! It also means that your bones are what you eat.

In the last chapter we saw how important it is that our bones have the support of a healthy gastrointestinal system that's able to (1) properly break down the food we eat, and (2) absorb the nutrients from the food. What do we mean by "nutrients"? Stated simply, nutrients are the substances our bodies need to be able to live, grow, and maintain good health. We require specific nutrients for the building and repair of our body's tissues, for the conversion of food to energy, to help maintain balance and proper functioning in all of our bodily systems and processes—and to preserve the health of our bones.

The quality of the food you take in is directly related to your bone density and overall bone quality. A diet that promotes bone health includes a range of whole foods that support the specialized bone cells (those osteoblasts and osteoclasts) that engage the bones in a continual process of renewal. Conversely, low-quality food or an imbalanced diet can lead to bone loss, because a poor diet deprives the bones of crucial nutrients.

Some of the nutrition questions I'm most often asked include:

o What is the best diet for maintaining bone health?

o Can I get everything I need from my diet?

o What supplements should I take, if any?

o What are the most important dietary changes I can make?

o Can diet alone reverse osteoporosis?

This chapter provides an overview of the most salient "do's and don'ts" related to diet, nutrition, and bone nourishment. You'll learn which foods are bone-building and which are bone-draining. We'll also take a look at the circumstances under which quality food might not be enough, who might be in need of supplements, and which supplements are the best for bone health. Although paying attention to nutrition is important across the lifespan, one might argue that it grows increasingly important as we age, when it becomes more difficult to develop and maintain bone mass. The good news is this: If you do the right things most of the time, your bones will benefit greatly.

First, the Basics: All the Macronutrients in the Right Amounts

As suggested above, although our bones need high-quality, nutrient-rich food, they also need a range of nutrients, and those nutrients need to be present in the right amounts and the right proportions. In other words, it's not enough to eat nutritious food—it's also important to make sure that your diet consists of the right balance of proteins, fats, and carbohydrates (the macronutrients), and to avoid eating too much or too little on a regular basis. An optimal diet includes sufficient protein, lots of vegetables and fruits, and good fats. And let's not forget the importance of water and other fluids, which even your bones need.

Before we look at the macronutrients in more detail, first let's determine *how much* food you should eat for optimal health and well-being. This question is often answered in terms of calories. The number of calories needed to maintain a given weight depends on a person's activity level. For example, someone who weighs 115 pounds and engages in a moderate level of physical activity will need approximately 2,000 calories each day to maintain their weight.

How do you determine what weight is appropriate for your size? If you are either overweight or underweight, you raise your risk for a range of health problems. A body mass index (BMI) calculator—

available on the Internet (see Resources)—is another useful tool, one that can help you assess whether your weight is where it should be. Be aware, however, that BMI recommendations can be misleading. Although they are based on height and weight, they do not take muscle size into account. Muscular strength is a key factor in fracture prevention. Many of my osteoporosis patients have a low body mass index, which means they could benefit from gaining weight, preferably in the form of muscle. If you're trying to lose weight, be sure your desired weight is appropriate for your size and that the weight loss does not include a decrease in muscle mass.

Protein

Ideally, protein should be a part of every main meal or snack. Consuming protein whenever you eat carbohydrates helps you avoid the insulin spikes that cause the "sugar crash" that can occur after you eat.

For adult women and men, the RDA (Recommended Dietary Allowance) for protein is 46 and 56 grams per day, respectively, a recommendation that does not take into account body weight, height, or activity level. Another recommendation states that daily consumption should amount to ¼ to ½ gram of protein per pound of body weight. A person weighing 140 pounds, for example, would consume 35 to 70 grams of protein each day. Yet another recommendation states that daily protein intake should amount to 20 to 30 percent of total caloric intake. That is the recommendation I tend to follow, and for most people it's a good yardstick.

And what about the source of your dietary protein? Some studies have shown that a diet with a high ratio of animal-based protein to vegetable-based protein results in increased fracture rates and bone loss. But the research on protein and bone health can be misleading. Some Americans do consume high amounts of protein. For example, if you typically eat eggs and bacon for breakfast, a burger with cheese for lunch, a soda, and a huge steak or perhaps a meat-and-cheese pizza for dinner, your diet is inflammatory (see below) and therefore not good for your bones or heart. On the other hand, although some experts theorize that meat is especially acidic and that excessive meat intake can lead to more calcium being excreted through the urine, the fact is that our bones *need* protein. If we don't get enough, the bones will suffer. Dietary protein increases circulating levels of insulin-like growth factor 1 (IGF-1), which, as you learned in Chapter 8, plays an important role in bone formation and maintenance. And contrary to the picture that's painted in many epidemiological studies of the average American, I find that many of my patients who have osteoporosis are deficient in protein.

Bottom line: Make sure you are consuming the right amount of protein, and get the majority of your protein from plant sources such as beans, legumes, nuts, and seeds. I also recommend limiting your intake of animal proteins to mostly lean meats and fish and deemphasizing red meat and dairy.

Fats

Despite what some diet gurus have told us in the past—namely, that fat is bad for you—dietary fats are essential to the health of the body. Cell walls, including those of the nerves and the brain, are made of lipids (fats). Fats are crucial for the proper functioning of the body and should comprise 20 to 35 percent of your caloric intake.

The best fats are the omega-3 fatty acids found in oily fish (e.g., salmon, sardines, mackerel), plant foods such as flax, chia, and hemp seeds, and some sea vegetables. The typical American diet, by contrast, is loaded with the omega-6 fatty acids found in vegetable, seed, nut, and bean oils; whole foods such as eggs and poultry; and processed foods such as cereals, bread, cookies, and cakes. The body requires some omega-6 fatty acids, but for Americans the average ratio of omega-6 to omega-3 fats is 12:1 or higher. The ratio should be 1:1 to 1:4; a ratio of 1:1 or 1:2 is optimal. One four-year study of fifteen hundred men and women showed that a high ratio of omega-6 to omega-3 fats in the diet is associated with lower bone density at the hip in both sexes.

If you read the labels of supplements containing omega-3 oils you'll notice the letters "EPA" (eicosapentaenoic acid) and "DHA" (docosahexaenoic acid), which are two types of omega-3 fatty acids. I typically recommend a minimum daily intake of 1,200 IU and 800 IU, respectively. Of course, some people need more or less depending on their health status and their diet.

Can too much fat be bad for you? Of course it can! Especially when it's low-quality fat. The worst fats are the manmade saturated "trans fats," for example, those contained in shortening, margarine, and other fats used to fry foods commercially. Although trans fats (technically named "trans fatty acids") naturally occur in small quantities in some foods, when they are manufactured, the process involves converting a liquid vegetable oil to a solid fat—mostly to lengthen shelf life. Ingredients that contain the words "hydrogenated" and "partially hydrogenated" are manmade trans fats. Animal-derived saturated fats (contained in butter, beef, pork, etc.) should also be minimized. Coconut oil is a saturated fat that in the past was considered unhealthy. In fact, recent studies have concluded that coconut oil is a heart-healthy fat.

Bottom line: Reduce your intake of "bad" fats, especially from fried foods, and increase your intake of fish and of seeds from the chia, flax, and hemp plants.

Carbohydrates

Generally speaking, food that is not fat or protein falls into the carbohydrate category (although there are some foods and dishes that combine the three macronutrients). As your body converts the food you eat to energy, it works first with the carbohydrates, which are the body's most easily digested fuel source. Carbs have gotten a bad rap over the years, but, like fats, carbs come in good and bad forms.

So far in this section we've learned that 20 to 30 percent of our caloric intake should consist of protein and another 20 to 30 percent should come from fats. If we do the math, this means that 40 to 60 percent of our caloric intake should consist of carbohydrates. I find, however, that it is best to keep the carbs between 40 and 50 percent of caloric intake and adjust fat and protein consumption accordingly.

Most of us know that sugars are simple carbohydrates. Sugars occur naturally in many foods, especially fruits. If you're looking to identify sugars on a food label, know that any ingredient containing the suffix "-ose" is a sugar. Fructose (fruit sugar), high-fructose corn syrup (condensed corn sugar), sucrose (sugar cane), dextrose, and maltose are all sugars that are often added to packaged foods.

We often speak of carbohydrate digestion as a process in which complex carbs are broken down into simple sugars and then absorbed into the bloodstream. The complex carbs found in whole foods are better for us than simple carbs, because complex carbs take longer to digest, meaning the resulting sugars enter the bloodstream more slowly, which is typically a good thing. Certainly, dietary sugars enter the bloodstream quickly, and other processed carbs also break down quickly. The more refined or processed the carbohydrate, the more rapidly it breaks down into sugar. Processed flours, especially white or rice flour, are speedily digested and then released as sugar into the bloodstream. Another example is "quick" or "instant" oatmeal. Whereas quick oatmeal rapidly turns into sugar, the less-processed steel-cut oats take more time to digest. Other complex carbohydrates that take longer to digest include whole grains, nuts, seeds, legumes, vegetables, and fruit.

When it comes to carbs, reading labels is a good way to keep from overdoing it. Be aware that the "total carbohydrate" number includes carbohydrates, fiber, and added sugar, so if you're trying to figure the net grams of carbohydrate in a food, subtract the grams of fiber—and keep in mind that everything in this net total will ultimately break down into a sugar of one kind or another. Keep in mind, too, that 4 grams of sugar is the equivalent of 1 teaspoon of sugar—so if the food you're consuming contains 28 grams of sugar per serving, you're ingesting 7 teaspoons of sugar! (Of course, whole foods such as un-processed meats and fish, as well as fresh fruits and vegetables from the produce department, don't carry food labels. Whole foods should form the bulk of your diet. Do an Internet search to find websites that list calorie and macronutrient data for whole foods.)

Bottom line: Remember that vegetables and fruits are whole-food sources of carbohydrates. Complex carbs (e.g., those contained in ap-ples, leafy greens, nuts, and seeds) are better for you than simple carbs (e.g., white rice, cookies, crackers, rice cakes, and sugary drinks—in-cluding fruit juices).

Hydration

Many of us know that hydration is crucial for good health. Fluids are absolutely essential for the elimination of toxins, the absorption and transportation of nutrients, the regulation of body temperature—and many other processes. Clearly, the health of one's bones depends on the overall health of one's body, and the body, which is approximately 60 percent water, needs lots of fluids to function as it should.

Generally speaking, if you live in a moderate climate and get limited exercise, the amount of fluids you should consume daily is approximately half your body weight in fluid ounces. By this logic, then, if you weigh 150 pounds, you would consume at least 75 ounces of fluids per day (8 fluid ounces equals one cup). The exact amount, of course, depends on factors such as your geographical location, whether or not you perspire heavily, your activity level on any given day, and whether you consume foods that deplete the body's fluids.

We hear or read different advice regarding how much fluid we need to consume. One extreme view is that we can get enough fluids just from the food we eat. But the Institute of Medicine has determined that an adequate intake (AI) for men is about thirteen cups of total beverages a day, while the AI for women is about nine cups of total beverages a day. My experience with patients is that most are not consuming enough fluids.

So what do we mean by "fluids"? When it comes to hydrating your body, the drinks that count the most are water and herbal teas. Caffeine and alcohol are dehydrating to some degree, but so are salt and sugar. Sugary drinks and fruit juices should be avoided or limited. Carbonated water (mineral water, for example) can be high in salt, so it's best to consume only one serving per day. One of the best liquids to consume during a meal is plain filtered water with fresh lemon or lime juice. The citrus juice aids digestion. *It is also important to know that you can consume too much water, which can lead to electrolyte imbalances—so be careful not to overdo it, either.*

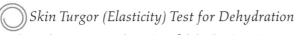 *Skin Turgor (Elasticity) Test for Dehydration*

Poor skin turgor can be a sign of dehydration. You can test the elasticity of your skin by pinching the skin on the back of your hand. Your skin should bounce back once you release it—if it doesn't, you may be dehydrated. (In the elderly, the best areas to test are the skin over the sternum and on the forehead.)

Cooling the Flames of Inflammation

Later in this chapter we'll talk about specific micronutrients (vitamins and minerals) that are essential for bone, but before we do, let's take a brief look at the type of diet you should *avoid*.

Are you eating an inflammatory diet? If so, ***DUMP THE JUNK!***

Everyone has experienced inflammation, which is a natural and necessary part of the body's response to injuries and to pathogens such as viruses and unwelcome bacteria. The swelling that occurs after injury to a muscle or joint is an inflammatory response. So is the redness and pain that flares up around a cut or abrasion. Inflammation has many causes; besides the normal inflammatory responses described above, certain chronic disease states are characterized by inflammation, for example, rheumatoid arthritis (RA). Some inflammatory conditions, including RA, are known to contribute to bone loss, *partially as a result of the inflammatory process itself.*

Inflammation is a helpful thing in small doses. During an infection it generates extra heat in targeted areas of the body, which creates an unsuitable temperature for pathogens. After a workout, inflammation in the muscles alerts the body to help reinforce broken-down muscle fibers and to deliver extra nutrients to rebuild a stronger muscular system for future workouts. However, inflammation also comes with harmful by-products, such as various acids that result from the inflammatory process. If these by-products are cleared from your body quickly, they are not harmful. But if the inflammation becomes a whole-body or chronic state, these acids and toxins can begin to affect your body in a negative way. It's a vicious circle. Constant inflammation creates an acidic state in the body, and constant acidity increases bodily inflammation.

Russell Greenfield, MD, who studied under Andrew Weil, MD, states that inflammation plays a much greater role in certain diseases than was once thought to be the case. Any word with the suffix "-itis" points to inflammation, which includes many well-known health conditions—for example, arthritis, appendicitis, and dermatitis. But Greenfield points out that illnesses such as cardiovascular disease, certain cancers, and Alzheimer's disease may be triggered in part by inflammation. On the flip side, some research indicates that type 2 diabetes triggers inflammation in the body. As we learned in Chapter 9, inflammation also plays a role in the pathogenesis of food sensitivities and food allergies. Because regular consumption of low-nutrient, high-sugar, processed foods (e.g., breads, cakes, cookies) can ultimately lead to inflammatory diseases, one of the main contributors to chronic inflammation may be the foods we eat.

There are lab tests that can help determine whether inflammation is occurring systemically in the body. However, some inflammatory conditions, for example, celiac disease (see Chapter 9), cannot always be detected with lab work. For our purposes, it is important to understand that when active bone loss is occurring it may be connected to an inflammatory process—one that is either diagnosable or flying under the radar. Generally speaking, some inflammatory processes can be significantly reduced or even resolved with a healthy anti-inflammatory diet, attention to any gastrointestinal conditions that may be occurring, and exercise. I always recommend an anti-inflammatory diet to my osteoporosis patients, especially those with active bone loss. Some ideas for lessening the inflammatory impact of your diet are outlined below.

Balance Acid and Alkaline Foods

Some health experts believe that an important aspect of an anti-inflammatory diet is making sure that it's high in alkaline foods and lower in acid-forming foods. All day long your body carefully manages and balances the degree to which your system too is acidic (acidosis) or, in rarer cases, too alkaline (alkalosis). According to the acid/alkaline theory, because chronic acidity is inflammatory, one of the most important things you can do for your bones is to limit your intake of acid-producing foods. The Standard American Diet (SAD) is replete with acid-forming foods—too high in meats and processed foods like flours, alcohol, sugar, and dairy products, all of which produce an acidic by-product in the body. Although almost all vegetables and most fruits can be considered "alkaline" foods, even some healthy foods are acidic. Beans are one example; however, dishes that include beans typically also include other ingredients—such as garlic, onions, or tomato (yes, tomato actually produces an alkaline by-product in the body)—that balance the acidity.

Acidity/alkalinity (alkalinity is also termed "basicity") is measured in terms of pH, which can be assessed in the blood and urine. A low pH means acidity, whereas a higher pH indicates alkalinity. Blood pH is tightly regulated, and the acid/base theory of health holds that if the system is too acidic the quickest way for the body to solve the problem is to increase the bones' osteoclastic activity, which releases calcium to buffer the excess acid. (It's important to point out that not all health experts agree with this hypothesis.) As you'll see below, some alternative doctors test the urine pH as a means to check systemic pH. To be on the safe side, eat a diet that tends toward alkaline-producing foods. If the scale tilts to the acidic side most of the day, every day, for years on end, bone loss may result.

Here are some tips for an anti-inflammatory eating plan, including increasing the diet's alkalinity:

o Add more alkaline foods to your diet when you can. You can find lists of alkaline-/acid-forming foods online, including my website. You will note that meat, sodas, sugar, coffee, alcohol, and refined carbohydrates (such as those found in cookies, cakes, and other sweets) are high acid formers. Some of the highest alkaline-forming foods are lemons, limes, parsley, kelp, kale, broccoli, and pumpkin seeds.

o Eat several servings of vegetables, especially green leafy vegetables, each day, as well as some fruits. Get plenty of raw foods in your diet. Eating a salad each day loaded with raw veggies is a good way to start. You also might want to add a fresh apple cider vinegar dressing to your salad—see my website for recipes.

o Get plenty of omega-3 fatty acids, such as those found in fatty fish, fish oil supplements, ground flax, chia, and hemp seeds, and walnuts.

o Eliminate trans fats and fried foods.

o If you eat animal protein, rely on fish and lean meats, such as chicken or turkey; cut back on red meat and dairy. (*Note:* There is growing concern about both fish toxicity and the sustainability of popular fishing methods. The Environmental Working Group, www.ewg.org, and the Monterey Bay Aquarium, www.montereybayaquarium.org, can help you identify which fish are safe to consume and which are best to avoid. See Resources.)

o Use fresh spices. Turmeric, ginger, and other spices can have an anti-inflammatory effect.

o Eat gluten-free—if not all of the time, then most of the time. Many people are sensitive to gluten, and many others have celiac disease, which means they're completely gluten intolerant. Celiac disease causes malabsorption and bone loss; if you have this condition you must view gluten as poison and avoid it entirely.

o Learn to cook using low heat. Visit my website for ideas, including delicious bean recipes for slow cookers.

Testing Your Urine pH

Some integrative and alternative doctors use a urine test to determine whether a patient's urine pH is too acidic, on the assumption that if the system is too acidic the body will go after bone to buffer the excess acid. There is certainly evidence that excessive sugar or meat intake creates an acidic ash in the body. On the other hand, as is the case with most health practices, views can be extreme, and there can be exaggeration as to what a test reveals and what you should do about it. I do think that the urine pH test provides helpful information. If your morning urine pH is too acidic on a regular basis, it most likely means that dietary changes are in order.

How to test urine pH: pH paper can be purchased in a health food store, online, or in a pharmacy. The test is graded using numbers and color. Make sure the paper is numbered consecutively (for example, 2-3-4-5) and doesn't skip numbers (for example, 2-4-6-8). Once you wet a strip with urine it will take only seconds to produce a number that corresponds with a color. Test your first void of the morning for seven days; document the number and then take the average over the seven days. A pH of 6.5 to 7 is best. If you are lower than 6.5 on a consistent basis, your urine is too acidic. You can change the pH of your urine by using the tips in the section above. Also check the pH of the water you drink. Water should have a pH of 7 or higher.

Minimize Your Toxic Load from Food and Other Sources

We all know that in our modern world we are exposed to many toxins. They come from sources ranging from the air we breathe to the furniture in our homes, to the lead in paint still found in older homes, to certain chemicals in our food and water supply. The good news is that many of us can minimize the toxins we are exposed to. We can start by doing our best to purchase foods with minimal contaminants. Following are some tips:

o *Pesticides:* As we saw in Chapter 8, some pesticides can disrupt our hormones, so it's best to avoid them whenever possible. Some organic foods strictly prohibit the use of any synthetic pesticides; however, most are grown with only minimal use of synthetic pesticides. The Environmental Working Group has on its website a list of the "dirty dozen" vegetables and fruits that contain high levels of pesticide residues (www.ewg.org/food news/summary.php). It's best to eat only organically grown versions of these foods. (The EWG also provides a list of the safest nonorganic foods.)

o *Mercury:* Mercury consumption is strongly linked to fish consumption. Varieties of fish that contain significant amounts of mercury include king mackerel, marlin, shark, swordfish, tilefish, orange roughy, and tuna. Visit the Natural Resources Defense Council's website (see Resources) for up-to-date information about which fish to avoid and which are safe to consume.

o *Lead:* Over 90 percent of any lead you may be exposed to can end up in your bone, which ultimately leads to poor bone health. Research conducted in 2013 found that some hot sauces imported from Mexico had a high lead content. Lipstick may contain lead (some women apply lipstick twenty times a day!), and some calcium and herbal supplements have also been found to contain high levels of lead. Always buy supplements from reputable sources (see Resources for a list of supplement providers that I recommend). The highest risk of lead exposure is still from paints produced prior to 1970. The EPA's website offers some good information on reducing your environmental lead exposure (see Resources).

o *Other heavy metals*: Lead and mercury are the most common metal contaminants, but it's also possible for other metals to enter the body, whether through ingestion or other exposure. Arsenic, cadmium, and chromium are among the metals that can be identified through lab work if contamination is suspected. (The human body requires small amounts of chromium; however, it has recently been discovered that certain hip replacement materials can cause toxic exposure to this metal.)

If you suspect that you or a loved one might have heavy metal exposure, you can be tested. There are several ways to test, including blood and hair analysis. You will find a list of labs that specialize in testing for heavy metal toxicity (see Resources).

The Osteo All-Stars

At this point you may be saying to yourself, "Okay, I appreciate the reminder that we should eat a balanced diet and avoid the junk, but aren't there *specific* nutrients that are really good for my bones? Tell me about those!" To be healthy, the bones need the many different nutrients found in a well-rounded, whole-foods diet, but certain nutrients are essential to bone health. This section and the next one describe some of the best bone-building vitamins and minerals, beginning with what I like to call the "osteo all-stars": calcium, magnesium, vitamin D, potassium, and vitamin K-2.

For each of the nutrients listed, I've included both the RDA and the therapeutic range commonly used by many practitioners, including me. Some people may require more or less of a particular nutrient depending on their specific needs; those who need the upper end of the therapeutic range are often individuals who have a malabsorption problem (see Chapter 9). Keep in mind that both the RDA and the therapeutic recommendations take into account all dietary sources— that is, from both foods and supplements. Note also that the dietary sources listed include herbal supplements.

Because it's all too easy to get too much of a good thing, please consult your health-care practitioner before you begin taking supplements. Supplements can have side effects, and they can have adverse interactions with prescription medications. Dietary supplements should be taken only under the supervision of a nutrition-savvy health-care provider.

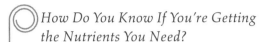

How Do You Know If You're Getting the Nutrients You Need?

If you're not sure you're getting the nutrients you need, you can keep a diet diary (available on my website to download). Once you've recorded your food intake for several consecutive days, search online for one of the great websites and/or apps that can help you see if what you're eating fits with your nutritional goals. Although nutrient-tracking tools can never be exact—because the specific quantity of a nutrient in a food depends, for example, on the serving size and on the quality of the soil in which it was grown—they provide good ballpark figures that can guide you in your intake of both macronutrients (fat, protein, carbohydrates) and micronutrients (vitamins and minerals).

Calcium

- *Recommended levels:* RDA 1,000–1,200 mg; therapeutic range 1,000–2,000 mg
- *Good dietary sources:* Dairy (especially yogurt—one of the best), collard greens, kale, bok choy, sardines with edible bones, bone broth made using organic poultry, salmon, beans, stinging nettle, oatstraw, blackstrap molasses, algae (add to soups)
- *Supplements:* Calcium citrate is absorbed more easily than some other sources, including calcium carbonate.

Calcium, probably the best-known bone-building mineral, is critical for bone; over 99 percent of the calcium in the body is stored in the bones. Hydroxyapatite, the main component of bone, is made primarily of calcium and phosphorus.

There is considerable controversy and misinformation related to calcium consumption, especially calcium supplementation. And there is concern that too much calcium can contribute to atherosclerosis (arterial plaque) in the heart and elsewhere. How do you know whether you're getting enough calcium—or possibly too much? The rest of this subsection addresses that question as well as some other FAQs about calcium.

Am I Getting Enough Calcium?

As you can see from the list below, the factors that contribute to calcium deficiencies are fairly wide-ranging. Some of them include:

o *Diet:* A dairy-free diet may or may not include sufficient calcium from other food sources.

o *Body size:* Small-framed people often eat small food portions, and smaller food portions contain fewer nutrients than larger food portions. Small-framed people may have insufficient calcium intake simply because their food intake is limited. Most people with osteoporosis are small people with small bones.

o *Digestive conditions:* Hypochlorhydria (low stomach acid) and malabsorption conditions especially pose risks for calcium deficiency. We need stomach acid to absorb calcium, and malabsorption conditions inhibit our ability to take in nutrients of all kinds.

o *Some over-the-counter and prescription drugs:* Prolonged use of medications that neutralize stomach acid (e.g., Tums, Pepto-Bismol) or inhibit stomach acid production (e.g., Nexium, Prilosec, Prevacid) can contribute to calcium deficiency by interfering with its absorption.

o *Surgical removal of the part of the small intestine that absorbs calcium or vitamin D:* For a visual representation of where in the small intestine calcium is absorbed, see Figure 9.2 on page 202.

o *Certain food components:* Some food substances interfere with calcium absorption, including phytates (found in whole grains, beans, nuts, and especially soy) and oxalates (discussed below). Many of these foods are good for you; however, if you consume a lot of them, you won't be absorbing as much calcium.

What about Oxalates?

Certain calcium-rich foods also contain oxalic acid, or oxalate, which renders some of the calcium in the foods unavailable for absorption by the body. Spinach is an example; other foods containing high amounts of oxalates include almonds, sesame seeds, beets, Swiss chard, and rhubarb. With the exception of rhubarb (which is especially high in oxalates), it's still good to include these foods in your diet. Although the body won't absorb all of the calcium contained in spinach, for example, spinach contains other nutrients, such as magnesium, that are good for bones. Basically, the message is this: Familiarize yourself with the high-oxalate foods; if you eat them, make sure your diet contains other calcium-rich foods that are *not* high in oxalates. Cooking does not significantly lower a food's oxalic content.

Am I Getting Too Much Calcium?

It depends. Generally speaking, the people who ingest too much calcium are those who consume significant amounts of dairy and/or take high doses of calcium supplements. Look beyond dairy for your calcium sources, and limit your dairy intake to no more than one to two servings each day. (The best dairy to consume is plain, organic, low-fat yogurt, which also contains natural probiotics that are crucial for digestive health.) Finally, if you take calcium supplements, make sure that the amount you're taking is appropriate for you and your bones.

Overdosing on Calcium? Barbara's Story

Barbara, who was receiving treatment for osteoporosis from her primary care physician, came to see me because she was experiencing chronic constipation and anxiety. She also had heart palpitations, muscle pain, and muscle cramping in her lower legs that was so severe she found it difficult to walk. Now sixty-three, Barbara had been diagnosed with borderline osteoporosis five years earlier. Although she had always been very fit (she ran thirty miles per week when she was younger) and although with the exception of her age she had no additional risk factors and no history of fractures, her diagnosis frightened her, so she was faithful in complying with her doctor's recommendations—which were to increase her vitamin D and calcium intake by 5,000 IU and 1,500 mg, respectively. The calcium supplement, when added to the six or eight glasses of milk she drank each day, meant that Barbara's calcium intake amounted to approximately 4,000 mg daily!

My first steps with Barbara were to have her stop the cal-
cium supplement, adjust her food intake so that she was con-
suming only 1,200 mg of calcium each day, and add a magne-
sium supplement to balance her calcium. Calcium helps muscles
contract, and magnesium allows them to relax. I suspected that
Barbara's symptoms were caused by an overload of calcium
combined with a magnesium intake insufficient to balance
the calcium surplus. Once Barbara made these simple dietary
changes, her energy levels increased and her muscle pain and
heart palpitations stopped.

Barbara's story exemplifies a diligent, cooperative patient
who thought she was doing the right thing for her bones. When
it came to calcium, her attitude was the more the better. Un-
fortunately, this is not the case. Barbara suffered severe symp-
toms for years as a result of too much calcium and not enough
magnesium, but the good news is that the remedy was simple,
requiring only the balancing of her nutrient intake.

Will High Calcium Intake Cause Heart Disease?

Some studies have linked calcium supplementation with an increased
risk of heart disease. It is important to remember that when a study
looks at masses of average Americans, those masses do not necessarily include you. A typical American, for example, does not eat a
healthy diet. She or he tends to consume too much salt, sugar, meat,
and poor-quality fats, and too few vegetables and fruits. As described
earlier in this chapter, such a diet is inflammatory and can contribute
to bone loss.

Furthermore, over the last ten years more and more people have
become aware that they might be deficient in vitamin D. I agree with
this analysis. What does vitamin D do? One of the main things it
does is increase calcium and phosphorus absorption by as much as 50
percent. This could potentially be problematic, especially when dietary calcium is high and you're also consuming a lot of inflammatory
foods. When on top of this you also fail to balance your calcium intake
with appropriate amounts of magnesium, you're asking for trouble.

Again, though, if you're reading this book you may not be typical
of those in the studies on calcium and heart disease. In my experience,

some people with osteoporosis or low bone density either do not ingest enough calcium or they're deficient in vitamin D—and most are low in magnesium, too.

> ◎ *Nutrients and Bone Strength*
>
> For a more complete understanding of the relationship between nutrition and bone health, it's helpful to keep in mind that bone health, or bone strength, depends on bone quality, and that bone density is *only one part of* overall bone quality (albeit a significant part). As described in the first chapter, bone density is only one piece of bone strength—and both bone density and bone quality are impacted by the foods we eat. If you do not get enough calcium in your diet, for example, you can lose bone density, and it's easy to see how a loss of bone density could impact bone strength. On the other hand, it's also possible (but rare) to have fragile bones even while bone density is relatively normal—and this points to issues of bone quality. For example, regular tobacco use will reduce bone quality, even if bone density remains unaffected. And vitamin C deficiencies can lead to deterioration of the collagen that's needed to keep bones supple enough to absorb impact (bone flexibility is another aspect of bone quality). Bone strength is complex, and bone-building nutrients are those that contribute to overall bone quality, including but not limited to bone density.

Magnesium

- *Recommended levels:* RDA 400–420 mg; therapeutic range 400–800 mg
- *Good dietary sources:* Kelp, leafy greens (e.g., spinach), mackerel (avoid king mackerel), quinoa, brown rice, kidney beans, lentils, oatmeal, bananas, nuts, seeds (especially pumpkin seeds)
- *Supplements:* Like other supplements, magnesium supplements come in many forms. Two of the more absorbable forms are magnesium citrate and magnesium glycinate. Bathing in Epsom salts (magnesium sulfate) has been shown to increase magnesium blood levels, and when applied topically, magnesium

chloride raises the levels of magnesium in the blood. (*Note:* Oral magnesium can cause loose stools. On the other hand, when balanced with calcium, it can resolve constipation.)

Although we don't hear much about the mineral magnesium, it is essential for the proper growth and maintenance of bones and the proper functioning of nerves, muscles, and other parts of the body. Magnesium deficiency is a problem for a significant number of people. Deficiencies are caused by several factors, including magnesium-poor diets and the mineral-depleted soil in which much of our food is grown.

Carolyn Dean, medical doctor, naturopath, and author of *Magnesium Miracle,* points out that our bones need magnesium if they are to assimilate calcium properly. Calcium and magnesium should be consumed at a ratio of around 2:1. Those whose diets are low in magnesium may have a calcium/magnesium intake of 10:1 or higher. Calcium and magnesium often occur together in plants; for example, nettles and oatstraw have high levels of both minerals.

Vitamin D

- *Recommended levels:* RDA 200–600 IU; therapeutic range 1,000–4,000+ IU

- *Good dietary sources:* Fortified foods (e.g., orange juice, milk), eggs, some mushrooms, cod liver oil (which I do not recommend, as it contains excessive amounts of vitamin A, which can result in bone loss). Humans' main source of vitamin D is exposure to the sun. In general, food sources alone will not provide the vitamin D you need. (See my website, www.Lani Simpson.com, to learn how the sun's UVB rays produce vitamin D-3 in the skin.)

- *Supplements:* There are two forms of vitamin D supplements: vitamin D-3 (cholecalciferol) and vitamin D-2 (ergocalciferol). I recommend vitamin D-3, as it is more stable than vitamin D-2 and is what our body produces naturally through exposure to the sun. Most people need at least 2,000 IU each day, and some need much more; the amount you need depends on your sun exposure and on how much you're taking in from food sources.

Vitamin D is fat-soluble, so if you don't absorb fats well you can still be deficient even if you supplement. It's always best to get input from a vitamin D–savvy health-care practitioner prior to supplementation, and it's also a good idea to have your vitamin D level tested (but be sure you order the correct test; see Chapter 5).

As we saw in Chapter 8, vitamin D is crucial for bone health. Vitamin D-3 converts to the hormone calcitriol, which increases the absorption of calcium and phosphorus in the small intestine by a whopping 50 percent.

According to vitamin D researcher Dr. Robert Heaney, whom I interviewed, most people's bodies utilize 4,000 to 5,000 IU of vitamin D each day. Although our number one source of vitamin D is the sun, not all sunlight produces vitamin D. It is produced only by the (invisible) UVB rays, which are easily blocked by fog, smog, sunscreens, and even the earth's atmosphere. Because North America is at a higher geographical latitude, the UVB rays have to travel through more atmosphere to reach much of the continent, a journey that blocks many, if not all, of these beneficial rays. Most North Americans, especially those who reside north of latitude 37 (San Francisco on the West Coast and Richmond, Virginia, on the East Coast), cannot produce vitamin D during winter months through sun exposure.

Entire books have been written about vitamin D. As stated above, the best way to know whether you're deficient is to test your blood level. If you choose not to test, know that supplementation in the 2,000 IU range tends to be safe for most people. Again, though, if you have a medical condition or you're concerned about adding vitamin D to your diet, check with a knowledgeable health-care provider first.

Potassium

- *Recommended levels:* RDA 4,700 mg; therapeutic range 4,000–6,000 mg
- *Good dietary sources:* Dairy, seeds and nuts, potatoes (with skin), sweet potatoes, winter squash, beets, avocadoes, papaya, melons, bananas, prunes, beans (especially white beans), black rice,

amaranth, quinoa, dark leafy greens, dried apricots, salmon, mushrooms

- *Supplements:* Consider potassium supplementation carefully, especially if you're taking medications that impact your potassium level. Consult with your health-care practitioner before supplementing.

Generally speaking, the bones use potassium to neutralize bone-depleting metabolic acids. Studies have shown that a diet high in potassium is beneficial for bone; one study, for example, found that supplementation with potassium citrate (2,350 mg) improved both bone density and bone microarchitecture in the elderly. That is an impressive result!

Potassium-rich foods are also important for maintaining a proper level of alkalinity in the body. Unfortunately, it is difficult for most people to get the potassium they need through dietary sources alone. Dairy is high in potassium, but those who don't consume much dairy—or who don't consume much food—are at an especially high risk for depletion of this vital mineral.

It's easy to test the blood for potassium levels (see Chapter 5). A low potassium level, or hypokalemia, can lead to weakness, lack of energy, high blood pressure, muscle cramping, gastrointestinal distress, arrhythmia, and abnormal electrocardiograms. Common causes of hypokalemia include insufficient potassium in the diet, severe diarrhea, improperly managed diabetes, extremely low-calorie diets, excessive sweating, chronic alcoholism, vomiting, Crohn's disease, potassium-depleting medications and diuretics, and laxative use. Although most individuals tend not to get enough potassium, excessive potassium intake also leads to problems. In fact, either extreme can result in abnormal heart rhythms. Too much potassium in the blood (hyperkalemia) is most common in people who have kidney or adrenal disease; some medications can also cause high blood potassium levels.

One of the reasons why potassium made my osteo all-star list is because studies are increasingly showing the importance of potassium and bone health. If you think your intake of potassium may be low, consider reading the article on potassium available on my website.

Vitamin K-2 (Vitamin MK-7 and Vitamin MK-4)

o *Recommended levels:* no RDA; MK-7 therapeutic range 90–200 mcg, MK-4 therapeutic range 10–45 mg

o *Good dietary sources:* Vitamin MK-4 is found in small amounts in meat, butter, and egg yolks; MK-7 is found primarily in fermented foods. Natto, a fermented soy product, is one of the best dietary sources of MK-7; fermented cabbage (sauerkraut) and kimchi contain small amounts.

o *Supplements:* It's probably best to get your MK-7 in supplement form as this vitamin is not sufficiently available in most of the foods we eat. The supplemental source is typically derived from natto. Supplemental MK-4 is a synthesized product.

It may seem odd that a vitamin with no RDA would make my all-stars list. Yet more and more research is showing that vitamin K-2 benefits the bones, blood vessels, and other bodily tissues. Vitamin K-2 belongs to the vitamin K family, a group of fat-soluble vitamins. Vitamins K-1 and K-2 are two of the main subgroups that occur within the larger group, and vitamins MK-4 and MK-7 are two of the main nutrients belonging to the vitamin K-2 category (also known as menaquinones).

Besides being available in small amounts in animal products, vitamin MK-4 can be made in minute amounts by the bacteria that line the large intestine. MK-7, as mentioned, is found in some fermented foods. (Vitamin K-1, or phylloquinone, occurs in plants, especially green vegetables; it contributes to healthy blood clotting, among other benefits.)

The following excerpt is from an article that appeared in the March 2008 issue of *Life Extension Magazine* titled "Protecting Bone and Arterial Health":

> The Japanese long ago recognized the power of vitamin K2 to maintain or restore bone health. In certain regions of Japan, a staple dish called natto or fermented soybean, frequently eaten several times a week, is uniquely rich in vitamin K2. Recent scientific examination has pinpointed vitamin K2, and in particular vitamin K2 in the form of menaquinone-7 (MK-7),

the active ingredient in this popular eastern Japanese dish, as having a supportive effect on bone quality during osteoporosis treatment. People living in the Japanese regions where this dish is eaten have several-fold greater blood levels of vitamin K2 (MK-7), accompanied by less osteoporosis and bone fractures.

A two-year Japanese study found that vitamin K2 (MK-4) reduced the incidence of vertebral (spine) fractures by 52% in 120 patients with osteoporosis, compared with patients who did not receive this nutrient. The high dose used in this trial—as with most studies examining vitamin K2's effect on bone density—was 45 mg/day.

Dr. Kate Rheaume-Bleue, a naturopathic physician and author of *Vitamin K2 and the Calcium Paradox,* notes that K-2 is critical for bone. She supports the use of MK-7 supplements and claims that studies show that it stays in the bloodstream longer than MK-4, which is why a lower dose may be effective.

MK-7 may very well turn out to support bone health and reduce fracture risk; however, only MK-4 has been used as a treatment for osteoporosis. Studies on MK-4 have demonstrated a modest increase in bone density and a reduction in fracture risk. As of the writing of this book, MK-7 has not been shown to reduce fractures, but epidemiologic and animal studies point to its support of bone and heart health. In my practice I use both forms. Research on vitamin K-2 continues, so check in at my website for updates on this newest all-star.

Other Important Nutrients

Silica

- o *Recommended levels:* no RDA; therapeutic range 6–15 mg
- o *Good dietary sources:* Water (hard water), grains (hulls), horsetail, sugar beet, cane pulp, alfalfa, comfrey, nettles, beer, and coffee (though I would not rely on the last two as your main sources—sorry)

Silica plays a role in the firmness and strength of the body's tissues, and while it is not considered an essential nutrient, we know it is needed for bone strength. Silica is found in the arteries, skin, and eyes. It is also found in collagen, the main structural protein in connective tissue. Silica is easily lost during food processing.

Phosphorus

- *Recommended levels:* RDA 700 mg; therapeutic range 800–1,200 mg

- Good dietary sources: As a general rule, high-protein foods (dairy, red meats, poultry, fish, eggs) are also high in phosphorus. Grains contain phosphorus, but in a form that is less easily digested.

After calcium, phosphorus is the most abundant mineral in the body. The bones need phosphorus, but our phosphorus-calcium consumption needs to be in balance—a ratio of 1:1.

Phosphorus deficiencies are rare. You may be deficient if you have a malabsorption condition or maintain a vegan diet, and many medications can interfere with phosphorus absorption. It is more common to have excess levels of phosphorus in the system, especially if one eats processed foods and drinks sodas that contain phosphates. Those with kidney disease are usually put on low-phosphorus diets. Do not supplement with phosphorus unless you know your level is low and your doctor recommends it. (See Chapter 5 for information on phosphorus testing.)

Zinc

- *Recommended levels:* RDA 8–11 mg; therapeutic range 15–30 mg

- *Good dietary sources:* Meats, particularly lamb and beef, shellfish, and dark poultry meat; beans (pinto, chickpea, kidney); sesame and pumpkin seeds; oats; dairy (cheese and yogurt)

Zinc has been shown to stimulate bone formation and inhibit bone resorption. Depletion of zinc in the soil is one reason why some people are deficient. Zinc deficiency is fairly common, especially in children.

Manganese

o *Recommended levels:* RDA 1.8–2.3 mcg; therapeutic range 2–5 mcg

o *Good dietary sources:* Spelt, brown rice, chickpeas, spinach, pineapple, pumpkin seeds, tempeh, rye, and oats

According to researchers at the University of Maryland Medical Center, insufficient manganese intake can result in bone malformation. Most of us tend to get what we need from the foods we eat.

Copper

o *Recommended levels:* RDA 900 mcg; therapeutic range 1–3 mg

o *Good dietary sources:* Oysters and other shellfish, organ meats, whole grains, beans, seeds, and nuts

Copper deficiency has been linked to osteoporosis. Whereas some researchers point to the depletion of this trace mineral in our soils, others note that copper deficiency is rare.

Boron

o *Recommended levels:* No RDA; therapeutic range 3–6 mg

o *Good dietary sources:* Raisins, almonds, hazelnuts, dried apricots, avocado, walnuts, Brazil nuts, kidney beans, and dates

Many animal studies have examined the connection between boron and bone. One study found that boron supplementation can stimulate bone formation and inhibit bone resorption in osteoporotic rats, showing that this mineral may have a therapeutic effect against osteoporosis.

Vitamin C

o *Recommended levels:* RDA 75–90 mg; therapeutic range 500–5,000 mg

o *Good dietary sources:* Guava, red or green bell pepper, tomatoes, kiwi, orange, grapefruit, strawberries, Brussels sprouts, and cantaloupe

Vitamin C helps our bones maintain collagen, which supports bones' flexibility so they're better able to absorb impact. Multiple studies link high vitamin C intake to higher bone mass and lower fracture rates.

Vitamin A

- *Recommended levels:* RDA 700–900 IU; therapeutic range 3,000–5,000 IU
- *Good dietary sources:* Liver, eggs, fatty fish, paprika, yams, carrots, dark leafy greens, butternut squash, dried parsley, lettuce, dried apricots, and cantaloupe

Vitamin A plays an important role in bone growth and bone maintenance, but be careful! It can also increase osteoclastic activity, which in turn can lead to bone loss.

There are two sources of dietary vitamin A:

1. Active forms are immediately available to the body and are obtained from animal sources. These are known as retinoids and include retinaldehyde and retinol.

2. Precursors, also known as provitamins, must be converted to active forms by the body. They are obtained from fruits and vegetables containing yellow, orange, and dark green pigments known as carotenoids, the most well-known being β-carotene (beta-carotene).

Provitamin A has not been shown to cause bone loss. Supplement labels can be confusing because the active vitamin A forms and provitamins are often lumped together. If you have osteoporosis or low bone mass make sure that your supplements do not contain active vitamin A unless you know you need it. Provitamin A is converted in the liver to form active vitamin A. Some individuals, such as those who have liver or thyroid disease, do not convert the beta-carotenes well and may need to supplement with the active form.

Finally, some people use creams with high doses of vitamin A to treat acne, psoriasis, and other skin conditions. These may also have a negative impact on bone health if used for a long period of time.

Two food sources to be careful of are liver and cod liver oil, both of which I recommend avoiding on a regular basis due to their high vitamin A content.

Vitamin B-6, Folic Acid, and Vitamin B-12

Vitamin B-6

- *Recommended levels:* RDA 1.1–1.7 mg; therapeutic range 25–50 mg
- *Good dietary sources:* Rice and wheat brans, dried herbs, pistachios, raw garlic, liver, cold-water fish, sunflower seeds, sesame seeds, and blackstrap molasses

Folic Acid (Vitamin B-9)

- *Recommended levels:* RDA 300–400 mg; therapeutic range 800–1,000 mg
- *Good dietary sources:* Beef liver, boiled spinach, black-eyed peas, fortified breakfast cereals, rice, asparagus, Brussels sprouts, and leafy greens

Vitamin B-12

- *Recommended levels:* RDA 2.4 mcg; therapeutic range 1,000–2,000 mcg
- *Good dietary sources:* Shellfish, organ meats, cold-water fish, red meat, dairy, and eggs

Some studies have shown a relationship between osteoporosis/osteoporosis-related fractures and deficiencies in vitamins B-2, B-6, folic acid, and B-12. Yet the research is inconsistent. Earlier studies concluded that deficiencies in folic acid and vitamin B-12 led to elevated levels of homocysteine, which is a marker of inflammation and is also correlated with heart disease, but studies reported between 2012 and 2013 dispute some of those findings.

So where does this leave us with regard to the impact of the B vitamins on bone? Although taking them to lower homocysteine levels may not work in some cases, the new studies do not change the fact that vitamin B deficiencies are common, and the B vitamins are supportive of many bodily tissues, including bone tissue. For now, make sure you're getting your B vitamins.

In particular, vitamin B-12 deficiencies are especially common in the elderly as well as in those who consume a lot of fried foods. It can also be difficult for vegetarians and vegans to get adequate amounts of B-12 as it is primarily found in animal products. If you are deficient in B-12 and you have digestive symptoms that make it difficult to ingest this supplement, sublingual and injectable supplements are also available. There is some debate regarding whether or not fermented foods contain B-12. My take is that some fermented foods may contain a small amount; however, I would not rely on fermented foods for B-12.

Strontium

- *Recommended levels:* No RDA; therapeutic range (as strontium citrate) 680–800 mg
- *Dietary sources:* Seafood, whole milk, wheat bran, meat, poultry, and root vegetables

As we learned in Chapter 7, some alternative doctors use strontium citrate to treat osteoporosis. (Strontium is heavier than calcium and can replace the calcium in bone, where it can lead to "false" increases in bone density.) In Chapter 6 we learned that the synthetic osteoporosis drug strontium ranelate (Protelos) has been linked to heart problems. Strontium citrate may cause heart problems as well. We don't yet know whether long-term use of strontium results in reductions in bone quality, but it does have side effects, so be sure that you're well-informed before adding this mineral to your bone-health program. At this point I recommend against it; however, research is ongoing, and my recommendation may change in the future.

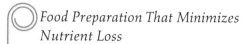 *Food Preparation That Minimizes Nutrient Loss*

Here are two food preparation tips that will maximize your food's nutrient value and also save you time: First, consider using a pulverizing blender (for example, a Vitamix) or juicer for preparing whole-food beverages and soups. Also, make use of a slow cooker (crockpot). Cooking with low heat, which is made easier by the use of a slow cooker, preserves nutrients. Check out the recipes on my website.

Supplement Savvy

When it comes to building and rebuilding bone, food should always be your first line of defense. Supplements are intended to provide nutritional support only when healthy food is not enough. They are *not* meant to compensate for a nutrient-deficient diet, especially a diet high in processed foods. There are some circumstances under which you may need supplements even if you eat a well-rounded, healthy diet. For example, most osteoporosis patients don't discover that they have the disease until they're well past age thirty—when their bones are no longer growing but instead are in the maintenance phase. In cases like these, in which a health condition is present, additional dietary reinforcements should be considered. Some of the main factors affecting whether or not nutritional supplementation is right for you include:

- *Digestive health:* You may need to supplement if you have a GI condition that limits your ability to access the nutrients in the food you eat.

- *Food intake:* The *amount* of food you eat may be insufficient to meet your nutritional needs, even if that food is nutritious. And certain diets may fail to provide all of the nutrients you need, or they may provide nutrients in excessive amounts—many diets are extreme. For example, the Atkins diet leans heavily on proteins and fats, while vegan diets provide no animal protein.

- *Food's growing conditions:* Depletion of the nutrients in our soils means fewer nutrients in the food that grows in those soils. In one study that compared nutrient data for foods from 1940, 1991, and 2002, of the seven minerals examined, all but sodium had undergone significant depletion by 2002; some minerals (e.g., copper) no longer occurred at all in the food.

Supplements are available from a large number of companies, and they vary widely when it comes to cost and quality—which can make it difficult to know which supplements to choose. Often, you get what you pay for, and quality is important. Good vendors provide supplements that come from high-quality, safe sources, and they also provide accurate labeling, so you can be assured that the ingredients and amounts you see on the bottle are what you're actually getting. But not all supplements are high-quality. Some contain fillers, and some contain low-quality nutrients that are less effective than higher-quality ones. And some supplements contain contaminants such as lead, pesticides, or other toxins.

Doctors who specialize in nutrition should be able to guide you to good supplement sources. The supplement vendors I buy from have their products evaluated and tested by third parties. See Resources for a list of reliable sources for supplements.

The supplements that I typically recommend for osteoporosis patients include a good multivitamin/-mineral that contains bone-essential nutrients such as boron, copper, zinc, and the B vitamins. Depending on a patient's test results, I also tend to prescribe vitamin D, as well as magnesium and calcium when they are needed. (Multivitamins usually contain calcium, magnesium, and vitamin D, too, so be sure to account for these nutrients before adding more.) My recommendations regarding other nutrients depend on each person's needs. Also, recommendations depend on whether someone is looking to prevent osteoporosis or whether he or she has been diagnosed with osteoporosis. Some individuals require additional vitamin K-1 and K-2, potassium, and the B vitamins; others may need additional protein or omega-3 fatty acids, or support for the adrenals and/or thyroid. Treatment with supplements is very individualized. Again, if you're considering supplements, it's always best to work with a knowledgeable practitioner to ensure that you're choosing what's best for you.

In addition to a high-quality multivitamin/-mineral and any other supplements your body requires, you may also want to consider milk basic protein, lactoferrin, whey powder, or probiotics.

- o *Milk basic protein, lactoferrin, and whey powder:* We learned about MBP and lactoferrin in Chapter 7, and we also learned that they can be overhyped. (Whey powder is another supplemental source of these milk-based proteins.) Don't expect any miracles if you have advanced osteoporosis, but know that each of these products has been shown to help stabilize bone markers, which demonstrates that they are likely benefiting the health of the bone. They may also increase bone density for some people. Those with dairy allergies or sensitivities may do okay with these products; however, if you have an allergy to dairy, consult with your doctor first.

o *Probiotics:* As we saw in Chapter 9, our gastrointestinal tract depends on the help of the many "good" bacteria that live in our intestines. More than five hundred different types of bacteria inhabit the small intestines. The body's natural bacterial balance can be compromised by a diet high in sugar and processed foods, an imbalance that can impede digestion. Probiotics are microorganisms that can help maintain proper levels of the "good" bacteria that occur naturally in the body.

Not surprisingly, probiotics come in supplement form, and they also occur in food. Food sources include yogurt, tempeh, natto, microalgae, honey, and fermented vegetables such as pickles, fermented cabbage (sauerkraut), and kimchi. Generally speaking, if a food is fermented, it contains probiotics. (There are also prebiotics, which are nutrients that feed probiotics. Foods that contain prebiotics include garlic, Jerusalem artichokes, asparagus, tomatoes, and bananas.) Cooking with low heat can help to preserve the probiotics that live in food; cooking with high heat destroys them.

Multivitamin/Mineral Basics

In addition to issues such as the quality of the ingredients in a supplement, another factor that impacts a supplement's effectiveness is the form it takes. As a general rule, one-a-day multivitamins are configured into a single, cement-like package that is hard to digest—and if you can't digest the vitamin pill, you can't absorb the nutrients it contains. The best multivitamins come in powdered, capsule form. You will be taking three to six capsules per day for the full daily dose, spread into smaller doses throughout the day. With larger doses, the body flushes any excess nutrients that enter the system; thus, splitting the daily dose increases the likelihood that more nutrients will be absorbed into the bloodstream. Finally, unless your doctor prescribes otherwise, be sure that your multivitamin does not contain vitamin A unless your doctor recommends it specifically (beta-carotenes are okay).

Nutrition Isn't Rocket Science—
You Can Revamp Your Diet Today!

This chapter provided a fair amount of detail related to the nutrients needed to maintain bone health. It also provided nutrition basics— because *the basics are well over half the battle.* It's helpful to know the details, but sometimes they can seem overwhelming, causing a person to feel that she or he can't possibly incorporate them into daily practice.

So don't let the details intimidate you! If your diet is balanced so that you're eating the proper amounts of the whole foods that provide proteins, fats, and carbohydrates; if you drink plenty of water; and if you avoid foods that are bad for your bones—you're well on your way to optimizing your bone health. As I've emphasized throughout this book, the most important bone-builders are a healthy gastrointestinal system that can properly absorb nutrients, solid nutrition, and physical activity that strengthens bones. We cover exercise in the next chapter.

 KEY POINTS FROM CHAPTER 10

o A balanced diet is critical for healthy bone quality and bone density.

o A pulverizing blender and a slow cooker are kitchen appliances that will help you prepare healthy, bone-supportive meals.

o Eat a diet that is rich in alkaline-producing foods to reduce inflammation.

o Too much vitamin A can result in bone loss.

o It can be difficult to get all of our nutritional needs met from the foods we eat.

o Supplements are often needed for patients with osteoporosis.

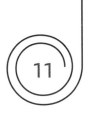

Strong Moves:
Exercise for Better Bones

"Don't just sit there! Do something!" This is what people say when they're in a panic. If you've been diagnosed with osteoporosis, you may well be feeling panicky—and even though you might be afraid that exercise could cause you to fracture a bone, the advice to "do something" is actually just what you need. Studies have shown that weight-bearing exercise improves bone strength, so a sedentary lifestyle is the opposite of what your bones need to be healthy.

There are many books for sale—and there are probably pamphlets in your doctor's office—that tell people with osteoporosis how to safely engage in physical activity. Most of them provide essential information to help patients with basic activities of daily living, for example, getting safely in and out of a chair, lifting heavy things without hurting oneself, or safely walking up and down stairs. Most advice of this sort is given to people who have a high fracture risk potential and may also have balance problems; it focuses on teaching patients how to avoid falls and fractures so they can maintain their physical independence. It may also describe basic exercise activities. Many of the readers of this book, by contrast, in addition to adhering to this essential advice, can also participate in a much more rigorous exercise program.

Remember the 1983 hit song "Break My Stride," by Matthew Wilder? "Ain't nothin' gonna break my stride / Ain't nothin' gonna slow me down / Oh no, I've got to keep on movin." A modified version of those lyrics can apply to people with osteoporosis. Whether you're a three-mile-a-day runner or confined to a wheelchair, movement is a key requirement for bone (and muscle) health. Ideally, and if you are able, you want to include weight-bearing exercises that are strenuous enough to give you a good workout while building new bone. Whether you've never worked out in your life or you're a natural athlete, this chapter shows you how to use physical activity to build and maintain bone health and prevent fractures. You also want to exercise safely, in a way that fits with your individual health status and physical limitations. As you read this chapter, please note that if you have been diagnosed with osteoporosis it is important for you to discuss your potential exercise restrictions with a health-care professional who knows and understands exercise as it relates to your individual case.

Why Exercise?

An active lifestyle that includes regular exercise benefits the body and mind immensely. Exercise improves digestion, hormone balance, metabolism, muscle tone, cognitive function, mood, and bone density. It boosts the metabolic rate, allowing the body to process food more efficiently. Through its impact on muscle strength and flexibility, exercise can also serve to support the bones. Consistent exercise develops proprioception, our sense of where our body is in space. Translated literally, "proprioception" means "sense of self." The proprioceptors are most abundant in our ankles, where they help us to avoid tripping and falling.

When you exercise regularly, you feel better. Workouts that use the body's full range of motions cause fresh blood to be circulated to all parts of the body. Good circulation allows the body, including the bones, to get the full benefit of the nutrition it takes in, and the fast-pumping heart helps the bloodstream cart away excess fluid, waste, and inflammatory by-products. Not only is exercise important for its own sake, but it's also necessary to offset the sedentary lifestyle led by many of us modern humans. Nowadays, whether at work or at home, most of us spend much of our time sitting, which makes deliberately engaging in physical activity more important than it was in centuries past.

For some readers it may feel like an impossible task to get to a place where exercise has a regular role in your life. Or perhaps your diagnosis has made you feel too frightened to continue your regular activities or to embark on an exercise program. However, if you are willing and able to make a consistent effort, physical activity can improve your bone health, reduce your risk of fractures—and enhance your health in many other ways as well.

Which Workouts Help Your Bones?

A regular exercise routine has been shown by the National Institutes of Health to prevent fractures by strengthening muscles and bones as well as improving balance, which helps reduce falling. In terms of *types* of exercise, we know that exercises that increase our heart rate—such as swimming, running, and biking—are good for the heart. But what are the best moves for building bone and maintaining bone mass? The answer, according to the National Osteoporosis Foundation, is weight-bearing exercise.

What exactly qualify as weight-bearing exercises? They consist of movements that make you work against the force of gravity while in a vertical position, and they fall into two categories: high impact and low impact. According to the NOF's website, high-impact weight-bearing exercises often require landing on your feet while performing activities such as dancing, running, hiking, jumping rope, tennis, or basketball. In contrast, although low-impact exercises may require your body to bear weight, they don't require you to lift yourself into the air. Examples of low-impact activities include elliptical machine workouts, low-impact aerobics, stair-step machine workouts, and walking, either on a treadmill or outside. Both low- and high-impact activities can help us maintain bone mass, but high-impact activities are especially beneficial because they stress the bones to some extent; bone-building occurs at a greater rate when the bones are stressed, or "impacted." Some studies have shown that a strong walking and hiking program may sustain bone density in certain parts of the body. A significant walking program that includes walking up some hills has been shown to maintain bone density in hips. However, walking has not been shown to benefit spinal bone density.

Perhaps the most compelling evidence of the link between weight-bearing activity and bone growth was discovered by the space program, when it was observed that astronauts who were exposed to decreased gravity conditions for long periods were losing bone density at an alarming rate. Identifying this condition, which is called space flight osteopenia, was the first time a strong connection was made between weight-bearing and bone density. Studies have shown that the average loss of bone density sustained by astronauts is 1 to 2 percent per month. The discovery of this "antigravity" problem has led to limits on the time astronauts are allowed to spend in space.

What Type of Exercise Is Right for You, and Where Do You Begin?

Before you take up any workout program, there are questions to ask about your physical abilities and the types of activities that are the best fit for you. Some of the factors to consider highlight where you are in terms of your bone and muscle health. Even if you have osteoporosis, that means different things for different people. A fifty-eight-year-old woman with borderline osteoporosis and no history of fractures is at a much lower risk of fracturing than a seventy-five-year-old man with severe osteoporosis and very poor muscle strength.

So where are you with your bone health? Have you suffered a low-trauma fracture? Do you feel fragile? Do you feel strong? Do you still have a bit of hop to your step? Do you have issues with balance? Are you already actively engaged in sports or exercise activities? If you participate in sports or exercise classes, have you had personal instructions and training? If not, are you willing to get the training you need?

If you're a sixty-year-old woman in great shape, you eat a nutrient-rich diet, and you've been diagnosed with borderline osteoporosis but have no other risk factors, you'll likely be able to shape and maintain a robust exercise program that includes high-impact exercises. Conversely, for many people with osteoporosis, it is likely that a long-term sedentary lifestyle has been one of the factors that have contributed to the condition. And some individuals may never have learned any exercise basics. If that's the case, to immediately begin engaging in an exercise program may be unsafe and can actually result in soft tissue injuries, stress fractures, or worse.

If you have been diagnosed with low bone density or osteoporosis, please see a physical therapist who specializes in osteoporosis before beginning any exercise program.

It is also a wise idea to apply the basic tenets of safe exercise. You should end your workout when you start to experience mild to moderate muscle discomfort. Ideally, you should only experience mild muscle soreness for twenty-four hours following working out. As your endurance develops, getting to your discomfort point will require you to exert more effort; you'll need to work out harder to exhaust the muscles. If you're not sure what "healthy" discomfort feels like, or if you feel unstable, it is best to work out with a trainer or partner who can assist you if necessary.

Here are some additional points to think about when exercising or contemplating taking up a new type of workout:

- *Posture:* You can think of poor posture as an accident happening in slow motion. If you are often hunched over your computer or you're constantly using your smart phone with your head craned forward, your body will start complaining over time. Many of us have poor sitting and standing posture, which leads to strained muscles, joint problems, and spinal misalignment. Poor posture can be a recipe for disaster if you're engaged in physical activity. Good posture is *the* starting point for *any* activity. If you're not sure whether your posture is good or poor, I highly recommend that you see a chiropractor or other health professional who can work with you on your posture. Even if you are hunched over because you have sustained one or more fractures in your spine, it is still important to maintain the best posture you can.

When it comes to protecting the spine while exercising, the importance of proper posture cannot be overstated. As we learned in Chapter 1, compression fractures of the spine are the most common fractures. Heavy pressure on the vertebral bodies (see Chapter 1 for diagram), even through improperly executed stretching, can result in spinal fractures in susceptible individuals. For example, when stretching the back of the legs you should not round the back; doing so puts stress on the vertebra. Instead, bend from the hips.

Gym Madness: Don't Injure Yourself Out of the Game

If you know what you're looking for when you're at the gym, you can see some of the most ineffective and injury-prone workouts imaginable. It's common to see treadmill walkers leaning on the rails or draping themselves over the front of the machine so that their lower body isn't fully engaged. And I see some of those same folks walking more slowly on the treadmill than they walk to their car! It's also common to see men and women lifting weights improperly, for example by distorting their posture to "work around" or otherwise wrestle with a weight that's too heavy. Physical activity may get your heart rate up, but it will also hurt you if you don't use proper "body mechanics." Even when poor posture and poor body usage aren't severe enough to put someone on the sidelines, they will make his or her workouts less effective because they fail to work the body in the ways intended. If you elect to start a weight-training program you will need expert advice (training and feedback) regarding your program. Proper body mechanics are essential, especially if you have low bone density.

o *Balance:* Good balance means fewer falls. One study showed that students participating in tai chi—a slow-moving martial-arts practice that enhances balance—were able to significantly reduce their falls. Other great activities for enhancing and improving balance are qigong and yoga. Balance goes a long, long way toward reducing fracture risk.

o *Flexibility:* Flexibility will allow you to get more enjoyment out of whatever exercise program you choose. More important, flexibility is one of the keys to injury prevention. Muscles that are limber versus tight are less likely to tear. And bodies that have the range of motion that's necessary for a given movement are less likely to fall. Take a stretching class or visit a bookstore if you're unsure how to improve your flexibility; there are many good books on basic stretching techniques. If you're not very flexible, exercise bands can help you stretch safely, and because they offer resistance, they also provide a powerful workout.

- *Core training:* The strengthening of the torso and back muscles is an important foundational component of any effective exercise program. A strong core helps the rib cage to expand fully and the diaphragm to work with less effort during respiration. A strong torso also improves posture, helping a person achieve the proper positioning needed for weight training, yoga, daily movements such as lifting and reaching, and any other physical activity. A strong core helps with balance. Taking a core-strength class is a great way to get core training; you can also get instruction from a personal trainer. If you're not already familiar with it, one device you'll likely encounter if you take a core-strength class is the exercise ball. Ball exercises improve core strength and balance while limiting the risk of falling.

- *Strength training:* Strength training refers to any exercise that's designed to build muscle. When we think of strength training we often think of weight lifting, but isometric exercises are also a form of strength training. Isometric exercises are resistance exercises that don't involve movement of the part of the body you're exercising—for example, pushing against a stable structure such as a wall could serve as an isometric exercise that strengthens arm and chest muscles. Generally speaking, isometric exercises are safe and gentle.

Another form of strength training that's relatively gentle involves the "wearing" of weights that add resistance during activities like walking and running. I ask some of my patients to wear a four- to ten-pound weight vest as part of their walking or running program; doing so adds bone-healthy stress to the spine. However, talk with your doctor before using a weight vest to make sure the added weight is safe for you.

- *Jumping:* Jumping on the ground has been shown in studies to increase bone density. I highly recommend jumping for the right patients. You can see a video on my website that demonstrates how to jump for different levels of physical fitness. I typically recommend starting with light jumping for fifteen to thirty seconds. But before you begin, watch the video!

    Rebounders are small trampolines for jumping on. I have two rebounders and love them as part of my exercise routine.

They can be especially good for people who have knee or hip problems because a trampoline is more forgiving than hard ground. The best rebounders are ones that use bungee cords instead of steel springs. I especially like the JumpSport and the Bellicon brands. Both have rails (must buy separately) that can help you balance. The JumpSport has one that goes completely across the trampoline, adding both safety and versatility with exercises. Both companies supply videos for beginners. Will using these rebounders increase bone density? Studies are scant; however, I think it is a very good exercise to include in your program, and I do think it may be stimulating to bone.

○ *Yoga:* Yoga is an excellent weight-bearing exercise that includes postures to strengthen both the lower and upper body. Many yoga postures put weight on the arms, which is a very good thing, as the forearm tends to be one of the weakest parts of the body. Yoga affords two additional benefits: It improves balance, which reduces a person's risk of falling, and it develops mindfulness, the ability to be "present" or more fully aware—which can also reduce the risk of falling. Although there is no conclusive research showing that people can gain bone density if they practice yoga, the weight-bearing postures are most likely helpful.

There are many types of yoga, and they differ in terms of how much weight-bearing exercise they provide and how strenuous they are. One form of yoga that I can personally recommend is Iyengar yoga, which is a type of hatha yoga. I am partial to this form because, having gone through the training required to be certified as an instructor, I know that the instructor training is intensive, requiring at least two years of study. Among other things, the program includes anatomy classes taught by physical therapists or other qualified health professionals. Some instructors specialize in working with osteoporosis patients. But be aware that some postures are not suitable for certain people (see the list in the box to the right).

○ *The Feldenkrais method:* The Feldenkrais method is a system of gentle movements that promote flexibility, coordination, and body awareness. It is used to improve both physical movement and general well-being through "physical reeducation," or, in

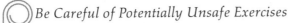

Be Careful of Potentially Unsafe Exercises

While it is true that any bone in the body can fracture when exercising due to a fall or some other mishap, some exercises pose a higher risk for people with osteoporosis. As we learned in Chapter 1, fractures of the spine are the most common fractures that people experience, especially as they get older. Therefore, when we engage in controlled exercise poses or routines—for instance, in yoga or strength training—it is vital to protect the spine. Following are some of the exercises that are not recommended for people who have a moderate or high risk for fractures:

- forward bending
- shoulder stands
- twists (rotational moves for the spine)
- jackknife (legs bent over the head)

slightly different terms, "somatic education." I highly recommend Feldenkrais for those who are new to exercise or have osteoporosis. Feldenkrais is an ideal practice for those who want to become more fully "present" in their bodies. Advanced athletes who want to minimize injuries also appreciate this program.

o *Pilates:* This is an exercise program that is focused on building strength, improving flexibility and balance, and preventing injury. It was initially created for rehabilitation, but was later adopted by dancers and athletes. Pilates is safe for most people who have osteoporosis. But for beginners, I recommend individual sessions that are supervised by trained teachers. Make sure your trainer works specifically with osteoporosis patients.

o *Exercise classes:* Can you do exercise routines at home, or do you need a supervised program? One of the biggest advantages to taking classes (or, better yet, hiring a personal trainer) is that with instruction you're likely to learn how to exercise properly so that you will get the most out of your workout and avoid injury. Some class instructors are highly trained and can help you with proper posture, and they'll also be able to suggest alternatives when you cannot complete a movement that's being demonstrated. (For example, many yoga instructors provide support tools such as poles or bolsters to help students for whom a particular posture is too difficult.) As mentioned earlier, however, if you have been diagnosed with osteoporosis, see a physical therapist before participating in exercise classes. Also, more and more classes are being offered for people who have osteoporosis or for those with limited abilities. Many YMCAs or senior centers offer such classes.

What if you can't afford to take an exercise class or hire a personal trainer? If you have osteoporosis, your insurance company may cover physical therapy. This can be a good alternative. Skilled physical therapists are able to design exercise programs that ensure a healthy, balanced workout. Also, visit my website for up-to-date recommendations on videos and books that you can use at home.

What about Pain?

Soreness after a workout is a sign that you have small tears in your muscle tissues. This is perfectly normal and in fact necessary. The body builds muscle through the process of repairing the muscle that's torn as a result of exercise. But there is an important difference between ordinary muscle soreness and a deeper level of pain that suggests injury. Soreness that lasts about twenty-four hours after a workout essentially lets you know you did some work, and that's a good thing; pain that impairs movement means you overdid it. One good way to avoid injury is to start slowly and see how your body feels the next day, adding to your program gradually over time.

For Athletes: Should You Consider Stopping a Sport or Activity Because You Have Osteoporosis?

"Okay," some of you are probably saying. "There are some helpful reminders here, but I've been active all my life. I like exercise, and I know how to do it properly. My question is, "Since my bones are vulnerable, do I need to stop?" This section will help you gauge whether you should continue your current activities or take up new ones. As it turns out, many activities can be continued safely if you modify them in ways that address your particular health status. Although you want to continue your active lifestyle, you also want to exercise the caution needed to avoid falls or other traumas that can result in fractures, joint damage, or worse. A key question to ask is how adept are you at the sport you love? For instance, if you've cycled all your life and you tend to ride safely, for you, cycling may be worth the risk of falling. On the other hand, if you're an older adult and you're active but not a cyclist, I'd advise you not to take up cycling now—whether or not you have low bone density.

The following strategies for injury prevention are especially relevant to those of you who are actively engaged in activities that give you lots of exercise:

o *Hikers:* Buy hiking poles! They are lightweight and they telescope to a small size, making them easy to keep on hand, and you can find them at most sporting-goods stores. Also, when hiking down steep hills, try walking sideways. This allows you to use more of your foot for balancing. Walking sideways down hills and using hiking poles can do a lot to keep you from sliding. You do not want to get caught on some slippery slope without poles for support and balance. If you do start slipping, it's better to get your pants dirty and slide down on your buttocks, if necessary, rather than risk falling on your hip.

o *Cyclists:* Keep up with the maintenance on your bike, and make sure it's the right size for your body. Go to a bike shop and have them adjust the seat and handlebars so you can ride comfortably. Check your tires regularly, and get new ones sooner rather than later. I suggest you use wider, mountain-bike tires. Get handlebars that allow you to sit upright rather than hunched over; improper neck alignment can cause spine damage. Be a defensive rider; observe what's happening at *every* corner. Drivers may be texting or doing something else that causes them to miss stop signs or fail to see you. Finally, use common sense. If you're not an experienced or stable rider your risk of falling and sustaining a serious injury is higher. I still ride, but I make sure to take side streets that have bike lanes and less traffic.

o *Runners:* To minimize falling, it's best to run in areas that have an even surface and no tripping hazards. It's also important to be sure that your shoes have the exact type of support you need. Have your gait analyzed by a trained professional. This will show you whether your feet and ankles roll inward (pronate) or outward (supinate) in a way that requires additional support so you can select shoes that minimize the risk of stress-related injuries to ankles, knees, or back. Shoe stores that specialize in running shoes often have staff who can analyze your gait and help you select the right shoes for you.

o *Yoga:* There are some postures in yoga that I consider too risky for those with osteoporosis. While those who have practiced for years should be able to maintain the postures with proper alignment, I have had more than one patient who has fractured bones doing yoga. Keep in mind that the older you are the more likely it is that certain postures can exert too much pressure for the body of the vertebrae to withstand; see box above for a brief list. Shoulder stands are generally too risky for those who've been diagnosed with osteoporosis. And unless the lumbar curve is maintained, forward bends also pose a high risk of injury to the spine when done incorrectly. Whether or not you have osteoporosis, it's always best to choose a form of yoga—and a yoga instructor—whose main focus is precision and the proper alignment of the entire body and spine. Iyengar yoga is an example of a precise, alignment-focused yoga form.

o *Snow skiing:* Downhill skiing poses a particularly high risk for hip fractures, so if you have osteoporosis you have to ask yourself if it's worth the risk. Cross-country skiing may be fine if your fracture risk is low and you're an experienced skier.

o *Tennis:* Although some tennis players use the sport for socializing, playing without much vigor, tennis can be a strenuous sport involving lots of running, jumping, and sudden side-to-side motion. If you've always been a strong player and you have just been diagnosed with osteoporosis, should you continue to play? Again, it depends on your risk for fracturing. To keep your bones safe, remember to be okay with letting some of those balls go.

o *Roller skating:* Some of you may have seen a video of me roller skating at age sixty. Even though I was an excellent and very experienced skater, I decided to hang up my skates when I turned sixty-three. As I'm sure you're aware, skating and falling can go hand-in-hand, and given my age and bone-health status I no longer consider skating worth the risk. As you might imagine, many of my colleagues were opposed to me skating and frankly I would advise others against skating.

Vibration Therapy

There's a whole lotta shakin' going on in the world of fitness. Dozens of companies sell vibration equipment, some of them promising development of muscle strength and loss of weight at a fraction of the time it would take with standard exercise. A selling point for many of the machines is that vibration also offers a potential noninvasive treatment for osteoporosis.

There are two main types of devices: those that deliver whole-body vibration (WBV) and those that deliver low-force or low-intensity vibration (LIV). Two companies make the low-intensity vibration machines: Juvent and Marodyne. Both products are based on Dr. Clinton Rubin's research. The LIV Tablet and the Juvent both impart what feels like a comfortable hum when you stand on them. By contrast, most WBV machines subject the user to an intense shaking. I worked with a master trainer using one such machine, the Powerplate. There was no question that my muscle tone built up quickly, but I never felt right about the intensity. My concern is that over time older adults could end up with conditions such as detached retinas, eye floaters, or even joint damage. For now I would steer clear of the WBV devices. I own a Juvent. It feels sturdy and seems like it will last a long time.

Multiple animal studies have demonstrated an increase in bone density using low-intensity vibration. One human study showed that postmenopausal women gained bone density, while the placebo group did not. The machines are expensive, so that will enter into your decision whether or not to purchase one. I have not used my Juvent long enough to know if I am increasing BMD. (I am also doing many other things to improve bone density, so isolating the effects of the machine will be tricky.) I stand on the Juvent for twenty minutes a day. It feels great, I know it won't hurt me, and it may very well help my bones.

Additional Safety Tips

Although this chapter is intended to get you exercising if you aren't already active, it's crucial that you choose activities based on your skill level and bone-health status. I've shared some tips that can help experienced athletic types continue their activities without injury. This section provides some additional safety pointers.

Whereas some injuries result from true accidents, exercise-related injuries often occur simply from errors in judgment. Take, for example, weekend warriors who sit all week long and are excessively active on the weekends. Or those who choose activities above their skill level, or who lack the balance, flexibility, or strength needed for the exercise they've chosen. And what about those who are injured because they used the wrong equipment, or the equipment they used was worn out or defective? Did you know that using the wrong equipment—or using improperly fitted equipment—is a major cause of injuries?

Following are some basic exercise-safety tips that can help keep your workouts injury-free:

o Work out regularly, not just on weekends. If you do choose to work out only on the weekends, take it easy. Your body may not be as "gung-ho" as your mind.

o Take lessons, or play it safe. If you aren't a natural athlete and don't have input from someone who is, don't attempt a rigorous run your first time out. Do something in your comfort range, or work with an experienced person who can help you keep yourself safe while still working hard enough to exhaust your muscles and challenging yourself to push your limits safely.

o Be careful on vacations. It is tempting while on holiday to try all sorts of activities you've never done before. Take care to avoid those that can put you in harm's way. For example, body surfing, water skiing, and parasailing are risky activities, especially if you're new to them. It may be difficult to hold back when the rest of your family or friends are eager to get on with the day's activities, but take the time to consider the risks before you participate.

o Wear proper clothing. Purchase the right shoes for the activity, and wear breathable attire that doesn't chafe. Proper clothing will go a long way toward making your workout comfortable and safe.

o Drink plenty of water. Adequate hydration is needed for proper muscle function. If you're not getting enough water, your risk for muscle injury is higher—and your exercise recovery time is longer. Staying well hydrated helps keep your muscles safe, and you won't need to rest as long between workouts.

o Eat some post-workout protein. When eaten soon after a workout, a dose of protein will help you build muscle. It may also help you build bone.

Most Important: Just Don't Fall!

When first diagnosing their patients with osteoporosis, doctors often place a great deal of emphasis on the following simple recommendation: *Don't fall!* This mostly sound advice is meant to change the way you view your normal activities, but it can also cause undue fear—or even terror.

As you've learned in previous chapters, there's a lot we can do to improve bone health and prevent fractures. Of course, one of the most important ways to prevent fractures is to avoid falling or some other mishap that can result in a broken hip, wrist, or vertebra. You learned in Chapter 1 that the overwhelming majority of hip fractures—90 percent or more—result from falling.

If you find yourself questioning your every movement, know that it is important to be *mindful* instead of *fearful*. Not only is fear a rather unpleasant emotional experience; even more important, it also causes physical tension, inhibiting the body from moving naturally and responsively, in the fluid way that's often required for reacting quickly to obstacles. Practicing mindfulness—a state in which you are relaxed yet focused—can help you stay aware of your surroundings while being centered in your body, so that you're less likely to lose your balance or trip over something in your path.

It may seem overly obvious to point out the importance of awareness and of paying attention to where you are stepping in order to avoid tripping and falling. But it's surprising how often people admit that they took a tumble because they simply were not paying attention. In our frenetic society it's easy to become preoccupied and distracted. When a lack of attention combines with the slower reflexes of older age and poorer eyesight, it becomes easier to fall.

If you feel especially vulnerable to falling—to the point where, even if you were in fact more aware of your surroundings, you would still feel unsafe—try this strategy: Before you start to move, think about where you plan to go, and be aware of the obstacles that lie between you and your goal. Then, plan your course—again, before you start to move. Be careful not to let this lead to paranoia. Too much focus on falling can become a fear-based, self-fulfilling prophecy.

Finally, the checklists below provide additional safety advice that can help you avoid a fall. These tips are taken from the National Institutes of Health publication *Once Is Enough: A Guide to Preventing Future Fractures*. For even more fracture-prevention tips, visit the NIH website at www.nih.gov.

Personal Safety Checklist

- Stay active to maintain muscle strength, balance, and flexibility.
- Have your vision and hearing checked regularly and corrected as needed.
- Discuss your medications with your doctor to see if specific medications (or medication combinations) make you more vulnerable to falling.

Indoor Safety Checklist

- Use nightlights throughout your home.
- Keep all rooms free of clutter, especially the floors.

○ Wear supportive, low-heeled, stable shoes, even at home. Avoid walking around in socks, stockings, or floppy slippers.

○ Keep floor surfaces smooth but not slippery. When entering rooms, be aware of differences in floor levels and thresholds.

○ Check that all carpets and area rugs have skid-proof backing or are tacked to the floor, including carpeting on stairs.

○ Keep electrical cords out of walkways.

○ Be sure that all stairways are well lit and that stairs have handrails on both sides.

○ Consider placing fluorescent tape on the edges of top and bottom steps.

○ Install grab bars beside tubs, showers, and toilets. If you are unstable on your feet, consider using a plastic chair with a back and nonskid leg tips in the shower.

○ Use a rubber bathmat in the shower or tub.

○ Keep a flashlight and extra batteries beside your bed.

○ Add ceiling fixtures to rooms that are lit only by lamps, or install lamps that can be turned on by a switch near the entrance to the room.

Outdoor Safety Checklist

○ In bad weather, consider using a cane, walking poles, or a walker for extra stability.

○ In winter, wear warm boots with rubber soles for added traction.

○ Look carefully at the floor surfaces in public buildings. Many floors are made of highly polished marble or tile that can be very slippery. When floors have plastic or carpet runners in place, try to stay on them whenever possible.

○ Use a shoulder bag, fanny pack, or backpack to leave hands free.

○ Stop at curbs, and check curb height before stepping up or down. Be cautious at curbs that have been cut away to allow access for bikes or wheelchairs. The incline may make you vulnerable to a fall.

Strong Moves: You Can Do It!

As you've learned in this chapter, "strong moves"—weight-bearing activities, especially high-impact activities—are vitally important to building and maintaining your bones. But whether regular exercise is new for you or not, if you have osteoporosis, you've probably wondered just how safe it is to exercise, as any physical activity is more likely to lead to falling than no activity at all.

The good news is that you *can* benefit your bones by exercising, because you *can* exercise safely—as long as the activities or sports you're involved in fit with your particular health status, which includes your risk for fractures.

Avoiding falls is important for everyone, and especially for those of us with low bone density. So while it is incredibly important to exercise, it's equally important to exercise in a way that minimizes fracture risk. If you're already active, this may mean altering (or even stopping) your favorite activity if it poses a high risk of falling. It also means that you have to be careful about trying new activities or sports in which you have little experience. For those who are new to exercise, decreasing your risk may mean taking classes or working with a trainer who can help you get started safely. And you'll always want to start slowly, building over time.

It *is* possible to work your muscles and your bones safely—even if your osteoporosis is advanced. This chapter provided a variety of safety tips that can help keep you on your feet while both getting the exercise you need and engaging in everyday activities.

Whether your fracture risk is low enough that you can continue with your ordinary activities safely—and perhaps try new ones—or if your osteoporosis requires you to be especially cautious, it's important to keep the following caveat in mind: As effective as exercise can be in building bone, it is not a solo cure. Remember, there are no magic bullets! Exercise will be most effective when you combine it with other healthy lifestyle choices that take into account the well-being of your whole body.

The two main lifestyle habits described in this book—exercise and diet—will be most helpful when they are, in fact, *habits*. Proper nutritional intake and exercise need to be a permanent part of your life, not just new behaviors you try for the short term. Any good that comes from temporary changes won't last, and a relapse to unhealthy habits will likely mean a return to many of the risk factors that caused your bone-health problems in the first place.

The good news, though, and the point I want to leave you with as you finish this book, is that *you can maintain and improve bone health and reduce your risk of fracturing a bone*. Although bone-building isn't easy and there are no quick fixes, the fact is most people can improve the health and quality of their bones, and some will be able to increase bone density. Studies have shown that certain nutrients are critical for maintaining bone density and sometimes can increase bone density, and that weight-bearing exercise can do so, too. Resolution of health problems that cause bone loss can help you develop healthy bone. I have seen many of my own patients stabilize bone loss and gain bone density. If you can make your quest to heal your bones a priority, you can slow or even stop bone loss—an endeavor that will provide significant benefit to the rest of your body as well.

 KEY POINTS FROM CHAPTER 11

○ Ninety percent of hip fractures occur following a fall.

○ Participating in balance exercises is important to reduce your risk of falling.

○ Low-vibration therapy is a good practice for many people with osteoporosis.

○ Muscle strength and flexibility are important for building and maintaining bone strength.

○ Avoid falls. Practice mindful movement while walking, exercising, and doing daily activities.

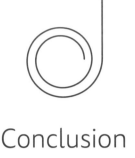

Conclusion

Given that you've decided to read a book on bone health, it's quite possible that you have been told you have a bone-health problem. And while it's true that I wrote this book to give hope and encouragement to those who have been diagnosed with osteoporosis, I also wanted to give all of my readers the information they need to build strong and supple bones at any age.

In this book I have laid out the multiple factors involved in proper bone-health assessment, along with the treatment options that are available for those who have been diagnosed with low bone density or osteoporosis. This book has shown you how to obtain an accurate bone density test and how to assess your own unique fracture risk. It has given you an overview of the factors that contribute to your particular bone-health status—along with the information that must be gathered for an accurate assessment of your bone health. It has provided an overview of both conventional and alternative osteoporosis treatments. And it has supplied information about the various factors that can slow bone loss or even prevent it from happening in the first place.

Most important, this book has offered you a way to think about bone that is more comprehensive and more accurate than the conventional perspective, which focuses almost entirely on testing for and treating low bone density. Bone health is much more than bone density alone. The overall strength of your bones depends on many factors, and keep in mind that if your *only* risk factor is low bone density, then your risk for fractures may be very minimal.

In fact, if you learn only one thing from reading this book, I hope it is this: There is no one-size-fits-all approach to bone health and the treatment of bone-health problems. Each of us is unique, and because bone health is complex and there are many different factors that can cause bone-health problems, every osteoporosis patient should be assessed on an individual basis. On the one hand, a diagnosis of osteoporosis should *never* mean an automatic prescription for medications. On the other hand, medications can prevent fractures and save lives when used in the right people who have a high fracture risk.

Although the current medical approach to treating osteoporosis is quite often one dimensional—prescribing medication, calcium, and vitamin D supplements—I've encouraged you to take the true complexity of bone into account, using an approach that, while it may or may not include medications, *always* includes proper nutrition; assessment for and resolution of any gastrointestinal dysfunction; hormone balancing if needed; and exercise. I've asked you to maintain a healthy skepticism regarding your diagnosis and the recommendations of your doctor(s), doing a good job on your homework before agreeing to any treatment program—and always watching out for treatments (conventional or alternative) that claim to be magic bullets!

Finally, as part of my attempt to give you an alternative and more integrative perspective on bone health, I've also emphasized the fact that, even if you have low bone density or osteoporosis, there is much you can do to reduce your risk for breaking a bone. Despite conventional medicine's focus on bone density as *the* diagnostic criterion for bone health—and on the use of medications that may slow bone loss in the short term—the real name of the game is fracture reduction. But as you've learned, not all of those with osteoporosis are in imminent danger of fracturing a bone, and there are risks associated with prolonged use of some medications that have been linked with an increased fracture risk.

The good news is that most of us can reduce our fracture risk. Bone health can be positively impacted at any time in life, if we choose to maintain a healthy, bone-building lifestyle that includes exercises to increase muscle strength and balance. And remember, there will always be new information, because bone-health research is ongoing. Be sure to check my website, www.LaniSimpson.com, for updates!

Appendix:
Bone Density Report

A *complete* bone density report includes a written report, scan pages and ancillary pages. Often, the doctor who ordered the test is sent only a two-page *written* report, without the scan pages. Ask the facility that conducted the bone density test to send the *entire* report to your doctor, including the scan pages (and the ancillary pages, which do not have pictures, but do have more diagnostic information). Also ask them to provide you with a complete copy for your own records. There are three companies that produce DXA machines: Hologic, General Electric (previously Lunar), and Norland. Each company has its own version of the diagnostic (scan) pages that form part of the report; however, they are all similar to the example pages that follow, "dummy" scans from Hologic.

As the example shows, the scan pages include diagnostic images (pictures of the area tested for bone density), which are necessary for a bone densitometrist to fully evaluate a patient's bone density test. If you plan to get a second opinion regarding your tests, make sure to obtain the scan pages for your most recent two (or, better yet, three) bone density tests. Some facilities (like Kaiser) will provide the report on a CD, which is fine. However, you or your doctor will need to be able to open the CD file to view and print the pages. For this purpose I use OsiriX, a free online application for uploading scan pages. Please note that *faxed* copies will not have the print quality necessary for proper analysis.

The most important areas of the body to test are the lumbar spine and the hip. A minimum of two areas should be scanned for diagnostic purposes, when possible. If you have had surgery on either your back or your hip (e.g., a hip replacement), the surgery site cannot be scanned. In such a case, the forearm should be scanned. The Vertebral Fracture Assessment (VFA) is not typically ordered. I order this test for patients who have been diagnosed with osteoporosis.

Although the scan pages from each company vary and can include eight or more pages, the most important pages to include are as follows:
- lumbar spine

- hip (femur bone) of one or both hips; sometimes both hips are included
- forearm
- ancillary pages for the hip and lumbar spine
- vertebral fracture assessment (VFA)

Note that on page 285 of the example pages below, we have pointed to the mathematical diagnostic information. Take a look at the headings. They may appear in a different order, depending on the DXA machine and the preference of the facility as to how they print their scan pages. Still, they can print exactly the information that is shown in the following scan pages. Quite often the area and bone mineral content (BMC) headings are not included. The minimal headings and numerical information that I require on the scan pages are the ones that appear below.

- Region: region of interest
- Area (cm²): area of bone selected (in square centimeters)
- BMC (g): bone mineral content (in grams)
- BMD (g/cm²): bone mineral density (in grams per square centimeter)
- T-score: applied to men and women over the age of fifty and post-menopausal women of any age
- PR (peak reference): your percentage compared to the average person of the same sex age twenty-six to twenty-nine
- Z-score: age-matched bone density score; used for men under age fifty and premenopausal women under age fifty
- AM (age matched): percentage of bone you have compared to a person of the same sex and age

Ancillary pages (pages 286 and 288) provide additional information—such as height and width of the vertebra selected—that some doctors find useful. You usually must ask specifically for the ancillary pages.

To see updates on bone density reporting or scan pages from other companies, visit my website: www.LaniSimpson.com.

Name: DOE, JANE	Sex: Female	Height: 66.0 in.
Patient ID:	Ethnicity: White	Weight: 120.0 lb
DOB: January 6, 1948	Menopause Age: 46	Age: 54

Referring Physician:

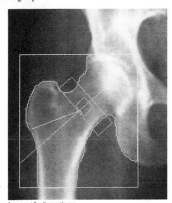

Image not for diagnostic use
k = 1.143, d0 = 52.5
94 x 105

Scan Information:

Scan Date: May 12, 2003
Scan Type: f Right Hip
Analysis: May 12, 2003 09:26 Version 11.2:3
         Right Hip
Operator: LH
Model: QDR 4500A
Comment:

DXA Results Summary:

Region	Area (cm²)	BMC (g)	BMD (g/cm²)	T - Score	Z - Score
Neck	5.08	2.99	0.589	-2.3	-1.4
Troch	10.47	6.05	0.578	-1.2	-0.6
Inter	20.18	16.76	0.831	-1.7	-1.3
Total	**35.73**	**25.80**	**0.722**	**-1.8**	**-1.2**
Ward's	1.22	0.61	0.494	-2.0	-0.4

Total BMD CV 1.0%, ACF = 1.043, BCF = 0.989, TH = 5.431
WHO Classification: Osteopenia
Fracture Risk: Increased

The **Neck** and **Total** rows of information are the only criteria used to assess bone density of the femur for determining a diagnosis.
The **Total** is an average of three areas: the femoral neck, intertrochanter, and trochanter. Ward's is not used for diagnostic purposes. The T-scores in this case indicate a diagnosis of low bone density (osteopenia).

Make sure your report includes all of the headings circled above in the DXA Summary. If the **Area** and **BMC** columns are not present, check for them in the ancillary page.

Total

BMD

Age

Reference curve and scores matched to White Female

Source: NHANES

Scanning machine company

HOLOGIC

Patient:	Doe, Jane	Facility ID:
Birth Date:	01/06/1941	Referring Physician:
Height / Weight:	63.5 in. 131.0 lbs.	Measured:
Sex / Ethnic:	Female White	Analyzed:

ANCILLARY RESULTS [DualFemur]

Region	BMD[1] (g/cm²)	Young-Adult[2,7] (%)	T-score	Age-Matched[3] (%)	Z-score	BMC (g)	Area (cm²)
Neck Left	0.892	86	-1.0	106	0.4	4.07	4.56
Neck Right	0.911	88	-0.9	108	0.5	4.05	4.44
Neck Mean	0.901	87	-1.0	107	0.4	4.06	4.50
Neck Diff.	0.018	2	0.1	2	0.1	0.02	0.12
Upper Neck Left	0.740	90	-0.7	113	0.7	1.66	2.25
Upper Neck Right	0.766	93	-0.5	117	0.9	1.67	2.18
Upper Neck Mean	0.753	92	-0.6	115	0.8	1.67	2.21
Upper Neck Diff.	0.026	3	0.2	4	0.2	0.01	0.07
Lower Neck Left	1.040	-	-	-	-	2.41	2.31
Lower Neck Right	1.050	-	-	-	-	2.38	2.26
Lower Neck Mean	1.045	-	-	-	-	2.39	2.29
Lower Neck Diff.	0.010	-	-	-	-	0.03	0.05
Wards Left	0.621	68	-2.2	94	-0.3	1.43	2.31
Wards Right	0.635	70	-2.1	96	-0.2	1.39	2.19
Wards Mean	0.628	69	-2.2	95	-0.2	1.41	2.25
Wards Diff.	0.014	2	0.1	2	0.1	0.04	0.12
Troch Left	0.630	74	-1.9	87	-0.8	8.89	14.10
Troch Right	0.628	74	-1.9	87	-0.8	8.47	13.48
Troch Mean	0.629	74	-1.9	87	-0.8	8.68	13.79
Troch Diff.	0.002	0	0.0	0	0.0	0.42	0.62
Shaft Left	1.047	-	-	-	-	13.97	13.34
Shaft Right	1.035	-	-	-	-	14.06	13.58
Shaft Mean	1.041	-	-	-	-	14.01	13.46
Shaft Diff.	0.012	-	-	-	-	0.09	0.24
Total Left	0.841	83	-1.3	97	-0.2	26.92	32.00
Total Right	0.844	84	-1.3	98	-0.2	26.57	31.50
Total Mean	0.842	84	-1.3	98	-0.2	26.75	31.75
Total Diff.	0.002	0	0.0	0	0.0	0.35	0.50

Note that the boxed rows of information correspond to the information on the scan page for the hip, and is the only criteria used to assess bone density of the hip for determining a diagnosis.

1 - Statistically 68% of repeat scans fall within 1SD (± 0.010 g/cm² for DualFemur Total)
2 - USA (Combined NHANES (ages 20-30) / Lunar (ages 20-40)) Femur Reference Population (v112)
3 - Matched for Age, Weight (females 25-100 kg), Ethnic
7 - DualFemur Total T-score difference is 0.0. Asymmetry is None.
   Filename: 54xb0n2sp9.dfx

Name: DOE, JANE	Sex: Female	Height: 66.0 in.
Patient ID:	Ethnicity: White	Weight: 120.0 lb
DOB: January 6, 1948	Menopause Age: 46	Age: 54

Referring Physician:

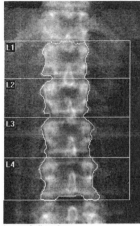

Image not for diagnostic use
k = 1.139, d0 = 49.9
116 x 145

Scan Information:

Scan Date:	May 12, 2003
Scan Type:	f Lumbar Spine
Analysis:	May 12, 2003 09:29 Version 11.2:3
	Lumbar Spine
Operator:	LH
Model:	QDR 4500A (S/N 45887)
Comment:	

DXA Results Summary:

Region	Area (cm²)	BMC (g)	BMD (g/cm²)	T-Score	Z-Score
L1	12.87	8.43	0.655	-2.5	-1.6
L2	14.32	11.50	0.803	-2.0	-1.1
L3	16.17	12.32	0.762	-2.9	-1.9
L4	18.39	14.27	0.776	-3.1	-2.0
Total	**61.75**	**46.52**	**0.753**	**-2.7**	**-1.7**

Total BMD CV 1.0%, ACF = 1.043, BCF = 0.989, TH = 5.803
WHO Classification: Osteoporosis
Fracture Risk: High

Note that the *Total* row of information is the primary criteria used to assess bone density of the spine for determining a diagnosis, when all four vertebra are of diagnostic quality. In this case, all four *are* of diagnostic quality, so the total represents the average of the four lumbar vertebra (L1-L4). The diagnosis in this case is osteoporosis, based on the *Total* T-score of -2.7.

Make sure your report includes all of the headings circled above in the DXA Summary. If the *Area* and *BMC* columns are not present, check for them in the ancillary page.

Total

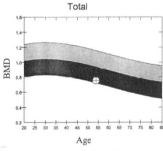

Age

Reference curve and scores matched to White Female

Source: Hologic

Patient:	Doe, Jane	Facility ID:
Birth Date:	01/06/1941	Referring Physician:
Height / Weight:	63.5 in. 131.0 lbs.	Measured:
Sex / Ethnic:	Female White	Analyzed:

ANCILLARY RESULTS [AP Spine]

Region	BMD[1] (g/cm²)	Young-Adult[2] (%)	T-score	Age-Matched[3] (%)	Z-score	BMC (g)	Area (cm²)	Width (cm)	Height (cm)
L1	0.830	73	-2.5	88	-1.0	10.43	12.56	3.7	3.36
L2	0.961	80	-2.0	94	-0.5	11.07	11.52	3.7	3.08
L3	0.936	78	-2.2	92	-0.7	12.27	13.12	3.9	3.35
L4	0.895	75	-2.5	88	-1.0	13.77	15.38	4.6	3.34
L1-L2	0.893	77	-2.3	91	-0.7	21.50	24.07	3.7	6.44
L1-L3	0.908	78	-2.2	92	-0.7	33.76	37.19	3.8	9.79
L1-L4	0.904	77	-2.3	91	-0.8	47.53	52.57	4.0	13.13
L2-L3	0.947	79	-2.1	93	-0.6	23.34	24.63	3.8	6.43
L2-L4	0.927	77	-2.3	91	-0.8	37.10	40.01	4.1	9.77
L3-L4	0.914	76	-2.4	90	-0.9	26.03	28.49	4.3	6.70

Lumbar ancillary pages are of particular importance for a densitometrist to parse out more specific information when needed. The bone density measurement is ideally based on an average of the measurements for four lumbar vertebrae, L1–L4. However, there are circumstances when all four vertebrae are not of diagnostic quality. One example is when surgery has been performed on one or more of the vertebrae, which should then be excluded from the diagnosis. If all four vertebrae are not of diagnostic quality, then three or even two can be averaged for the diagnosis, but never only one vertebra. The ancillary results allow the reporting doctor to select the proper diagnostic vertebrae. Refer to Chapters 2 and 3 for more information regarding selection of vertebrae.

1 -Statistically 68% of repeat scans fall within 1SD (± 0.010 g/cm² for AP Spine L1-L4)
2 -USA (Combined NHANES (ages 20-30) / Lunar (ages 20-40)) AP Spine Reference Population (v112)
3 -Matched for Age, Weight (females 25-100 kg), Ethnic
Filename: 54xb0n2sp9.dfx

Name: DOE, JANE	Sex: Female	Height: 66.0 in
Patient ID:	Ethnicity: White	Weight: 120.0 lb
DOB: January 6, 1948	Menopause Age: 46	Age: 54

Referring Physician:

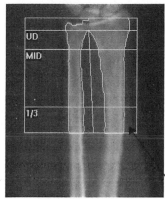

Image not for diagnostic use
k = 1.159, d0 = 67.6
180 x 91, Forearm Length: 24.0 cm

Scan Information:

Scan Date: May 12, 2003
Scan Type: a L.Forearm
Analysis: May 12, 2003 09:33 Version 11.2:3
Left Forearm
Operator: LH
Model: QDR 4500A (S/N 45887)
Comment:

DXA Results Summary:

Radius + Ulna	Area (cm²)	BMC (g)	BMD (g/cm²)	T - Score	Z - Score
UD	5.39	2.33	0.433	0.4	1.1
MID	11.10	6.42	0.578	-0.2	0.8
1/3	5.17	3.36	0.649	-0.6	0.4
Total	21.67	12.12	0.559	-0.1	0.9

Note that the boxed row is the only criteria used to assess bone density in the forearm for determining a diagnosis.

1/3 (Radius + Ulna)

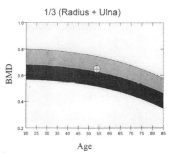

Age

Reference curve and scores matched to White Female

Source: Hologic

HOLOGIC

Name: Patient ID: Age:	Sex: Ethnicity: Date of Birth:	Height: Weight: Menopause Age:

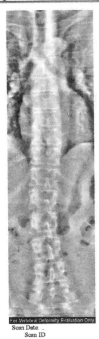 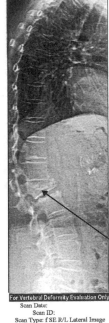

The vertebral fracture assessment allows a densitometrist or radiologist to check to see if there are any old or new fractures that are present in the thoracic and lumbar regions of the spine. The VFA cannot detect whether a fracture is recent or old. X-rays or other imaging tests may be needed to determine if a fracture is new.

Compression fracture of the spine.

These images were acquired from two different test subjects.

For Vertebral Deformity Evaluation Only
Scan Date..
Scan ID
Scan Type: f SE AP Image

For Vertebral Deformity Evaluation Only
Scan Date:
Scan ID:
Scan Type: f SE R/L Lateral Image

A spine fracture indicates 5X risk for subsequent spine fracture and 2X risk for subsequent hip fracture.

World Health Organization criteria for BMD interpretation classify patients as Normal (T-score at or above -1.0), Osteopenic (T-score between -1.0 and -2.5), or Osteoporotic (T-score at or below -2.5).

Vertebral Fracture Assessment (VFA)

This assessment is not typically ordered unless you have had a fracture or you have been diagnosed with osteoporosis. There are additional pages that are included with the VFA report and you can request a full copy of those pages as well. The most important scan page is the one you see here with the full spine images. The densitometrist will assess the images and check to see if you have any fractures in your spine. More information on this study can be found in Chapter 3.

References

Chapter 1

National Osteoporosis Foundation. "Learn about Osteoporosis." http:// www.nof.org/learn (accessed March 14, 2014).

American Academy of Orthopaedic Surgeons. "Hip fracture prevention." http://orthoinfo.aaos.org/topic.cfm?topic=A00121 (accessed March 15, 2014).

Fugh-Berman, Adriane. "A Bone to Pick with Bone Drugs." http://nwhn .org/print/473 (accessed March 15, 2014).

Rosen, Clifford J., and Mary L. Bouxsein. "Mechanisms of Disease: Is Osteoporosis the Obesity of Bone?" *Nature Clinical Practice Rheumatology* 2, no. 1 (2006): 35–43. doi:10.1038/ncprheum0070.

Perrien, D., N. Akel, E. Dupont-Versteegden, R. Skinner, E. Siegel, L. Suva, and D. Gaddy. "Aging Alters the Skeletal Response to Disuse in the Rat." *AJP: Regulatory, Integrative and Comparative Physiology* 292, no. 2 (2006): R988–96. doi:10.1152/ajpregu.00302.2006.

Nielsen, S. Pors. "The Fallacy of BMD: A Critical Review of the Diagnostic Use of Dual X-Ray Absorptiometry." *Clinical Rheumatology* 19, no. 3 (2000): 174–83. doi:10.1007/s100670050151.

Ott, Susan. "Osteoporosis." http://courses.washington.edu/bonephys /opop/opop.html#def (accessed March 15, 2014).

NIH Osteoporosis and Related Bone Diseases National Resource Center. "Glossary." http://www.niams.nih.gov/Health_Info/Bone/About_Us /Glossary.asp#O (accessed March 15, 2014).

National Institutes of Health. "The National Institutes of Health Consensus Development Conference Statement (March 27–29, 2000): Osteoporosis Prevention, Diagnosis, and Therapy." http://consensus.nih .gov/2000/2000osteoporosis111html.htm (accessed March 14, 2014).

NIH Osteoporosis and Related Bone Diseases National Resource Center. "What Is Osteoporosis? Fast Facts: An Easy-to-Read Series of

Publications for the Public." Last modified January, 2011. http://www
.niams.nih.gov/Health_Info/Bone/Osteoporosis/osteoporosis_ff.asp
(accessed March 15, 2014).

Ott, Susan. "Vertebroplasty and Kyphoplasty." http://courses.washington
.edu/bonephys/opvertebro.html (accessed March 15, 2014).

Khosla, S., L. Melton, M. Dekutoski, S. Achenbach, A. Oberg, and B. Riggs.
"Incidence of Childhood Distal Forearm Fractures Over 30 Years: A
Population-Based Study." *JAMA: The Journal of the American Medical
Association* 290, no. 11 (2003): 1479–85. doi:10.1001/jama.290.11.1479.

National Institutes of Health. "Why Are the Tween and Teen Years So
Critical?" Last modified January 4, 2010. https://www.nichd.nih.gov
/milk/prob/Pages/critical.aspx (accessed April 9, 2014).

U.S. Preventive Services Task Force. "Screening for Osteoporosis:
Recommendation Statement." Last modified January 2011. http://www
.uspreventiveservicestaskforce.org/uspstf10/osteoporosis/osteors.htm
(accessed March 15, 2014).

Department of Health & Human Services Administration on Aging.
"Projected Future Growth of the Older Population." http://www.aoa.gov
/Aging_Statistics/future_growth/future_growth.aspx#age (accessed
March 15, 2014).

Hamdy, Ronald, and Jennifer Culp. "Clinically Speaking: The Osteo-
porosis Report Card: Our Current Evaluation." *East Tennessee Medical
News.* http://www.easttennessee.medicalnewsinc.com/news.php?view
Story=1820 (accessed March 15, 2014).

Centers for Disease Control and Prevention. "Falls among Older Adults:
An Overview." Last modified September 20, 2013. http://www.cdc.gov
/homeandrecreationalsafety/falls/adultfalls.html (accessed March 15,
2014).

Lloyd, Janice. "Winter Falls, Bone Fractures May Point to Osteoporosis."
USA Today, January 8, 2013. http://www.usatoday.com/story/news
/nation/2013/01/04/health-bones-winter-osteoporosis/1764219 (accessed
March 15, 2014).

American Academy of Orthopaedic Surgeons. "Position Statement
1113: Osteoporosis/Bone Health in Adults as a National Public Health
Priority." Last revised September 2009. www.aaos.org/about/papers
/position/1113.asp (accessed April 20, 2014).

Kolata, Gina. "Study Finds Steady Drop in Hip Fracture Rates, but Reasons Are Unclear." *The New York Times*, August 25, 2009. http://www.ny times.com/2009/08/26/health/26hips.html?_r=1& (accessed March 16, 2014).

Leslie, W. D., S. O'Donnell, S. Jean, C. Lagace, P. Walsh, C. Bancej, S. Morin, D. Λ. Hanley, and Λ. Papaioannou. "Trends in Hip Fracture Rates in Canada." *JAMA: The Journal of the American Medical Association* 302, no. 8 (2009): 883–89. doi:10.1001/jama.2009.1231.

Stevens, J. A., and R. Anne Rudd. "Declining Hip Fracture Rates in the United States." *Age and Ageing* 39, no. 4 (2010): 500–503. doi:10.1093/age ing/afq044.

Wright, Nicole C., K. G. Saag, J. R. Curtis, W. K. Smith, M. L. Kilgore, M. A. Morrisey, H. Yun, J. Zhang, and E. S. Delzell. "Recent Trends in Hip Fracture Rates by Race/Ethnicity among Older US Adults." *Journal of Bone and Mineral Research* 27, no. 11 (2012): 2325–32. doi:10.1002/jbmr .1684.

Hayes, W. C., E. R. Myers, J. N. Morris, T. N. Gerhart, H. S. Yett, and L. A. Lipsitz. "Impact Near the Hip Dominates Fracture Risk in Elderly Nursing Home Residents Who Fall." *Calcified Tissue International* 52, no. 3 (1993): 192–98. doi:10.1007/BF00298717.

Vanasse, A., P. Dagenais, T. Niyonsenga, J. Grégoire, J. Courteau, and A. Hemiari. "Bone Mineral Density Measurement and Osteoporosis Treatment after a Fragility Fracture in Older Adults." *BMC Musculoskeletal Disorders* 6 (2005): 33. doi:10.1186/1471-2474-6-33.

Centers for Disease Control and Prevention. "Hip Fractures among Older Adults." Last modified September 20, 2013. http://www.cdc.gov /homeandrecreationalsafety/falls/adulthipfx.html (accessed April 9, 2014).

Chapter 2

Lewiecki, E. M., and L. Cerruto. "Case Study: Management of Poor Response to Bisphosphonate Therapy." http://www.projectsinknowledge .com/osteoporosis/osteoporosis_1/Case-Study-Management-Poor -Response-to-Bisphosphonate-Therapy.cfm?jn=1894.04 (accessed March 16, 2014).

U.S. Department of Health & Human Services. *Bone Health and Osteoporosis: A Report of the Surgeon General.* Rockville, MD: U.S. Dept. of

Health and Human Services, Public Health Service, Office of the Surgeon General, 2004. http://www.ncbi.nlm.nih.gov/books/NBK45513/ (accessed March 15, 2014).

Çetin, A., E. Özgüçlü, L. Özçakar, and A. Akıncı. "Evaluation of the Patient Positioning during DXA Measurements in Daily Clinical Practice." *Clinical Rheumatology* 27, no. 6 (2008): 713–15. doi:10.1007/s10067-007 -0773-0.

Ott, Susan. "Answer [Find BMD Interpretation Mistakes]." http://courses .washington.edu/bonephys/mis/ans18.html (accessed March 17, 2014).

Chapter 3

Blake, G. M., and I. Fogelman. "The Role of DXA Bone Density Scans in the Diagnosis and Treatment of Osteoporosis." *Postgraduate Medical Journal* 83, no. 982 (2007): 509–517. doi:10.1136/pgmj.2007.057505.

Lewiecki, Michael. *Mike's Manual (A Clinician's Guide to the Management of Osteoporosis, New Mexico Bone Densitometry Referral Codes).* Albuquerque, NM: New Mexico Clinical Research, 2003.

Ott, Susan. "T and Z Scores." http://courses.washington.edu/bonephys /opbmdtz.html (accessed March 17, 2014).

Schneider, Diane L. *The Complete Book of Bone Health.* Amherst, NY: Prometheus Books, 2011.

U.S. Preventive Services Task Force. "Screening for Osteoporosis: Recommendation Statement." Last modified January 2011. http://www .uspreventiveservicestaskforce.org/uspstf10/osteoporosis/osteors.htm (accessed April 9, 2014).

Spiegel, Alix. "How a Bone Disease Grew to Fit the Prescription." http:// www.npr.org/2009/12/21/121609815/how-a-bone-disease-grew-to-fit-the -prescription (accessed March 16, 2014).

Chapter 4

Schneider, Diane L. *The Complete Book of Bone Health.* Amherst, NY: Prometheus Books, 2011.

Foundation for Osteoporosis Research and Education. "10-Year Fracture Risk Calculator." Last modified December 2012. https://riskcalculator .fore.org/default.aspx (accessed April 9, 2014).

Brenner, J. "FRAX: A Brand New Tool for the Management of Osteoporosis." *Clinical Correlations: The NYU Langone Online Journal of Medicine* (2008). http://www.clinicalcorrelations.org/?p=818 (accessed March 16, 2014).

News-Medical.Net. "Strengths and Limitations of FRAX in Assessing Fracture Risk." Last modified August 3, 2011. http://www.news-medical .net/news/20110803/Strengths-and-limitations-of-FRAX-in-assessing -fracture-risk.aspx (accessed April 9, 2014).

International Society for Clinical Densitometry. "2010 Official Positions of the ISCD/IOF on the Interpretation and Use of FRAX in Clinical Practice." Last Modified January 4, 2003. http://www.iscd.org/official -positions/2010-official-positions-iscd-iof-frax (accessed April 9, 2014).

International Society for Clinical Densitometry. "Fracture Risk Models." Last Modified December 30, 2012. http://www.iscd.org/resources /fracture-risk-models (accessed April 9, 2014).

Chapter 5

Paley, L., T. Zornitzki, J. Cohen, J. Friedman, N. Kozak, and A. Schattner. "Utility of Clinical Examination in the Diagnosis of Emergency Department Patients Admitted to the Department of Medicine of an Academic Hospital." *Archives of Internal Medicine* 171, no. 15 (2011): 1394–96. doi:10.1001/archinternmed.2011.340.

Everson, C. A., A. E. Folley, and J. M. Toth. "Chronically Inadequate Sleep Results in Abnormal Bone Formation and Abnormal Bone Marrow in Rats." *Experimental Biology and Medicine* 237, no. 9 (2012): 1101–109. doi:10.1258/ebm.2012.012043.

Skugor, Mario. "Osteoporosis." http://www.clevelandclinicmeded.com /medicalpubs/diseasemanagement/endocrinology/osteoporosis-disease (accessed March 16, 2014).

Chapter 6

Spiegel, Alix. "How a Bone Disease Grew to Fit the Prescription." http:// www.npr.org/2009/12/21/121609815/how-a-bone-disease-grew-to-fit-the -prescription (accessed March 16, 2014).

Kelleher, Susan. "Disease Expands Through Marriage of Marketing and Machines." *The Seattle Times*, June 28, 2005. http://community.seattle times.nwsource.com/archive/?date=20050628&slug=sick28m (accessed March 16, 2014).

NPR. "Pillbox Biography: The Creation of a Blockbuster Drug." Last modified December 21, 2009. http://www.npr.org/templates/story/story.php?storyId=121585433 (accessed April 9, 2014).

Ott, S. M. "What Is the Optimal Duration of Bisphosphonate Therapy?" *Cleveland Clinic Journal of Medicine* 78, no. 9 (2011): 619–30. doi:10.3949/ccjm.78a.11022.

Singer, Natasha. "Drug Suits Raise Questions for Doctors, and Juries." *The New York Times*, November 10, 2010. http://www.nytimes.com/2010/11/11/health/11bone.html?pagewanted=all&_r=0 (accessed March 16, 2014).

Larson, Erik. "Merck Starts Fresh Trial on Fosamax Broken-Leg Claims." *Bloomberg,* April 7, 2013. http://www.bloomberg.com/news/2013-04-08/merck-starts-fresh-trial-on-fosamax-broken-leg-claims.html (accessed March 17, 2014).

Clarke, Toni. "FDA Panel Advises Calcitonin Salmon Not Be Used for Osteoporosis." *Reuters*, March 5, 2013. http://www.reuters.com/article/2013/03/05/us-fda-calcitonin-idUSBRE92418H20130305 (accessed March 17, 2014).

Lowry, Fran. "FDA Panel Says to Stop Marketing Salmon Calcitonin for Osteoporosis." *Medscape Medical News*, March 6, 2013. http://www.medscape.com/viewarticle/780323 (accessed March 18, 2014).

Schneider, Diane L. *The Complete Book of Bone Health.* Amherst, NY: Prometheus Books, 2011.

ADAM, Inc. "Osteoporosis: In-Depth Report." *The New York Times.* http://www.nytimes.com/health/guides/disease/osteoporosis/print.html (accessed March 17, 2014).

Green, J., G. Czanner, G. Reeves, J. Watson, L, Wise, and V. Beral. "Oral Bisphosphonates and Risk of Cancer of Oesophagus, Stomach, and Colorectum: Case-Control Analysis Within a UK Primary Care Cohort." *BMJ: British Medical Journal* 341 (2010). http://www.bmj.com/content/341/bmj.c4444 (accessed March 17, 2014).

Cardwell, C. R., C. C. Abnet, M. M. Cantwell, and L. J. Murray. "Exposure to Oral Bisphosphonates and Risk of Esophageal Cancer." *JAMA: The Journal of the American Medical Association* 304, no. 6 (2010): 657–63. doi:10.1001/jama.2010.1098.

National Osteoporosis Foundation. "Types of Osteoporosis Medications." http://www.nof.org/articles/22 (accessed March 17, 2014).

Smith, Michael. "ASBMR: Analysis Adds to Evidence of Unusual Fractures." *MedPage Today*, October 20, 2010. http://www.medpagetoday.com/MeetingCoverage/ASBMR/22859 (accessed March 17, 2014).

Brody, Jane E. "Revisiting Bone Drugs and Femur Fractures." *The New York Times*, March 7, 2011. http://www.nytimes.com/2011/03/08/health/08brody-bone.html (accessed March 17, 2014).

National Osteoporosis Foundation. *Clinician's Guide to Prevention and Treatment of Osteoporosis*. Washington, DC: National Osteoporosis Foundation, 2013. http://nof.org/files/nof/public/content/file/2237/upload/878.pdf (accessed March 17, 2014).

U.S. Department of Health & Human Services, Food and Drug Administration. "How Long Should You Take Osteoporosis Drugs?" Last Modified November 15, 2013. http://www.fda.gov/ForConsumers/ConsumerUpdates/ucm309688.htm (accessed April 9, 2014).

Bilezikian, J. "Osteonecrosis of the Jaw: Do Bisphosphonates Pose a Risk?" *New England Journal of Medicine* 355, no. 22 (2006): 2278–81. doi:10.1056/NEJMp068157.

"A 3-year Holiday from Bisphosphonates Appears Safe." *Cure*, April 19, 2011. http://www.curemagazine.com/index.cfm/fuseaction/news.show/NewsArticle/id/13/news_id/3139 (accessed April 15, 2014).

Watts, N. B., and D. L. Diab. "Long-Term Use of Bisphosphonates in Osteoporosis." *Journal of Clinical Endocrinology & Metabolism* 95, no. 4 (2010): 1555–65. doi:10.1210/jc.2009-1947.

Fujita, T., M. Fukunaga, A. Itabashi, K. Tsutani, and T. Nakamura. "Once-Weekly Injection of Low-Dose Teriparatide (28.2 μg) Reduced the Risk of Vertebral Fracture in Patients with Primary Osteoporosis." *Calcified Tissue International* 94, no. 2 (2014): 170–75. doi:10.1007/s00223-013-9777-8.

McCormick, R. Keith. *The Whole-Body Approach to Osteoporosis: How to Improve Bone Strength and Reduce Your Fracture Risk*. Oakland, CA: New Harbinger Publications, 2008.

Schneider, J. P. "Should Bisphosphonates Be Continued Indefinitely? An Unusual Fracture in a Healthy Woman on Long-term Alendronate."

Geriatrics 61, no. 1 (2006): 31–33. http://www.ncbi.nlm.nih.gov/pubmed /16405362 (accessed April 9, 2014).

Odvina, C. V., S. Levy, S. Rao, J. E. Zerwekh, and D. S. Rao. "Unusual Mid-shaft Fractures During Long-Term Bisphosphonate Therapy." *Clinical Endocrinology* 72, no. 2 (2010): 161–68. doi:10.1111/j.1365-2265 .2009.03581.x.

Edwards, B. J., A. D. Bunta, J. Lane, C. Odvina, D. Sudhaker Rao, D. W. Raisch, J. M. Mckoy, I. Omar, S. M. Belknap, V. Garg, A. J. Hahr, A. T. Samaras, M. J. Fisher, D. P. West, C. B. Langman, and P. H. Stern. "Bisphosphonates and Nonhealing Femoral Fractures: Analysis of the FDA Adverse Event Reporting System (FAERS) and International Safety Efforts." *The Journal of Bone and Joint Surgery* (American) 95, no. 4 (2013): 297–307. doi:10.2106/JBJS.K.01181.

Solomon, D. H., M. C. Hochberg, H. Mogun, and S. Schneeweiss. "The Relation Between Bisphosphonate Use and Non-Union of Fractures of the Humerus in Older Adults." *Osteoporosis International* 20, no. 6 (2009): 895–901. doi:10.1007/s00198-008-0759-z.

Foundation for Osteoporosis Research and Education. "New Drug Revolutionizes Osteoporosis Treatment." http://www.fore.org/resources /arnaud.html (accessed April 3, 2014).

Bodenner, D., C. Redman, and A. Riggs. "Teriparatide in the Management of Osteoporosis." *Clinical Intervention in Aging* 2, no. 4 (2007): 499–507. http://www.ncbi.nlm.nih.gov/pmc/articles/PMC2686338 (accessed April 9, 2014).

Chen, P., P. D. Miller, P. D. Delmas, D. A. Misurski, and J. H. Krege. "Change in Lumbar Spine BMD and Vertebral Fracture Risk Reduction in Teriparatide-Treated Postmenopausal Women with Osteoporosis." *Journal of Bone and Mineral Research* 21, no. 11 (2006): 1785–90. doi:10.1359/jbmr.060802.

Watanabe, A., S. Yoneyama, M. Nakajima, N. Sato, R. Takao-Kawabata, Y. Isogai, A. Sakurai-Tanikawa, K.Higuchi, A. Shimoi, H. Yamatoya, K. Yoshida, and T. Kohira. "Osteosarcoma in Sprague-Dawley Rats after Long-term Treatment with Teriparatide (Human Parathyroid Hormone (1–34)." *The Journal of Toxicological Sciences* 37, no. 3 (2012): 617–29. doi:10.2131/jts.37.617.

Subbiah, V., V. S. Madsen, A. K. Raymond, R. S. Benjamin, and J. A. Ludwig. "Of Mice and Men: Divergent Risks of Teriparatide-Induced Osteo-sarcoma." *Osteoporosis International* 21, no. 6 (2010): 1041–45. doi:10.1007/s00198-009-1004-0.

Watts, N. B., C. Roux, J. F. Modlin, J. P. Brown, A. Daniels, S. Jackson, S. Smith, D. J. Zack, L. Zhou, A. Grauer, and S. Ferrari. "Infections in Postmenopausal Women with Osteoporosis Treated with Denosumab or Placebo: Coincidence or Causal Association?" *Osteoporosis International* 23, no. 1 (2012): 327–37. doi:10.1007/s00198-011-1755-2.

Inkovaara, J., R. Heikinheimo, K. Jarvinen, U. Kasurinen, H. Hanhijarvi, and E. Iisalo. "Prophylactic Fluoride Treatment and Aged Bones." *BMJ: British Medical Journal* 3, no. 5975 (1975): 73–74. doi:10.1136/bmj.3.5975.73.

Dambacher, M.A., J. Ittner, and P. Ruegsegger. "Long-Term Fluoride Therapy of Postmenopausal Osteoporosis." *Bone* 7, no. 3 (1986): 199–205. doi:10.1016/8756-3282(86)90018-9.

Haguenauer, D., V. Welch, B. Shea, P. Tugwell, J. D. Adachi, and G. Wells. "Fluoride for the Treatment of Postmenopausal Osteoporotic Fractures: A Meta-Analysis." *Osteoporosis International* 11, no. 9 (2000): 727–38. doi:10.1007/s001980070051.

Loke, Y. K., R. Cavallazzi, and S. Singh. "Risk of Fractures with Inhaled Corticosteroids in COPD: Systematic Review and Meta-Analysis of Randomised Controlled Trials and Observational Studies." *Thorax* 66, no. 8 (2011): 699–708. doi:10.1136/thx.2011.160028.

Flores, Pam. "Interview with Dr. Jennifer Schneider on Spontaneous Femur Fractures from Osteoporosis Meds." *HealthCentral,* November 29, 2011. http://www.healthcentral.com/osteoporosis/c/76444/147539/spontaneous (accessed March 17, 2014).

Chapter 7

Chen, Y., C. Tseng, Y. Lo, R. Lin, C. Chen, G. Wang, M. Ho, and C. Tzeng. "Synthesis of Aminoalkoxy Substituted 4,5-Diphenylisoxazole Derivatives as Potential Anti-Osteoporotic Agents." *Medicinal Chemistry* 9, no. 5 (2013): 748–55. doi:10.2174/1573406411309050015.

Agnusdei, D., and L. Bufalino. "Efficacy of Ipriflavone in Established Osteoporosis and Long-Term Safety." *Calcified Tissue International* 61, no. S1 (1997): S23–27. doi:10.1007/s002239900381.

Bawa, S. "The Significance of Soy Protein and Soy Bioactive Compounds in the Prophylaxis and Treatment of Osteoporosis." *Journal of Osteoporosis* 2010 (2010): 1–8. doi:10.4061/2010/891058.

Toba, Y., Y. Takada, Y. Matsuoka, Y. Morita, M. Motouri, T. Hirai, T. Suguri, S. Aoe, H. Kawakami, M. Kumegawa, A. Takeuchi, and A. Itabashi. "Milk Basic Protein Promotes Bone Formation and Suppresses Bone Resorption in Healthy Adult Men." *Bioscience, Biotechnology, and Biochemistry* 65, no. 6 (2001): 1353–57. doi:10.1271/bbb.65.1353.

Aoe, S., Y. Toba, J. Yamamura, H. Kawakami, M. Yahiro, M. Kumegawa, A. Itabashi, and Y. Takada. "Controlled Trial of the Effects of Milk Basic Protein (MBP) Supplementation on Bone Metabolism in Healthy Adult Women." *Bioscience, Biotechnology, and Biochemistry* 65, no. 4 (2001): 913–18. doi:10.1271/bbb.65.913.

Xie, F., C. Wu, W. Lai, X.Yang, P. Cheung, X. Yao, P. Leung, and M. Wong. "The Osteoprotective Effect of Herba Epimedii (HEP) Extract in Vivo and in Vitro." *Evidence-Based Complementary and Alternative Medicine* 2, no. 3 (2005): 353–61. doi:10.1093/ecam/neh101.

Adami, S., L. Bufalino, R. Cervetti, C. Marco, O. Munno, L. Fantasia, G. C. Isaia, U. Serni, L. Vecchiet, and M. Passeri. "Ipriflavone Prevents Radial Bone Loss in Postmenopausal Women with Low Bone Mass over 2 Years." *Osteoporosis International* 7, no. 2 (1997): 119–25. doi:10.1007/BF01623686.

Alexandersen, P., A. Toussaint, C. Christiansen, J. P. Devogelaer, C. Roux, J. Fechtenbaum, C. Gennari, and J. Y. Reginster. "Ipriflavone in the Treatment of Postmenopausal Osteoporosis: A Randomized Controlled Trial." *JAMA: The Journal of the American Medical Association* 285, no. 11 (2001): 1482–88. doi:10.1001/jama.285.11.1482.

Rüegsegger, P., A. Keller, and M. A. Dambacher. "Comparison of the Treatment Effects of Ossein-Hydroxyapatite Compound and Calcium Carbonate in Osteoporotic Females." *Osteoporosis International* 5, no. 1 (1995): 30–34. doi:10.1007/BF01623655.

Chapter 8

Liu, J., H.Zhao, G. Ning, Y. Chen, L. Zhang, L. Sun, Y. Zhao, M. Xu, and J. Chen. "IGF-1 as an Early Marker for Low Bone Mass or Osteoporosis in Premenopausal and Postmenopausal Women." *Journal of Bone and Mineral Metabolism* 26, no. 2 (2008): 159–64. doi:10.1007/s00774-007-0799-z.

Sakuma, K., and A. Yamaguchi. "Sarcopenia and Age-Related Endocrine Function." *International Journal of Endocrinology* (2012): 1–10. doi:10.1155 /2012/127362.

Seifert-Klauss, V., and J. C. Prior. "Progesterone and Bone: Actions Promoting Bone Health in Women." *Journal of Osteoporosis* (2010): 1–18. doi:10.4061/2010/845180.

Pereira, R. M., A. M. Delany, and E. Canalis. "Cortisol Inhibits the Differentiation and Apoptosis of Osteoblasts in Culture." *Bone* 28, no. 5 (2001): 484–90. doi:10.1016/S8756-3282(01)00422-7.

Harvard Medical School. "What Are Bioidentical Hormones?" http:// www.health.harvard.edu/newsweek/What-are-bioidentical-hormones .htm (accessed March 17, 2014).

North American Menopause Society. "KEEPS Report: KEEPS Results Give New Insight into Hormone Therapy." http://www.menopause.org /annual-meetings/2012-meeting/keeps-report (accessed March 17, 2014).

Ohlsson, C., D. Mellström, D. Carlzon, E. Orwoll, Ö. Ljunggren, M. K. Karlsson, and L. Vandenput. "Older Men with Low Serum IGF-1 Have an Increased Risk of Incident Fractures: The MrOS Sweden Study." *Journal of Bone and Mineral Research* 26, no. 4 (2011): 865–72. doi:10.1002/jbmr .281.

Chau, K., S. A. Atkinson, and V. H. Taylor. "Are Selective Serotonin Reuptake Inhibitors a Secondary Cause of Low Bone Density?" *Journal of Osteoporosis* 2012 (2012): 1–7. doi:10.1155/2012/323061.

Manson, J. E. "The Kronos Early Estrogen Prevention Study." *Women's Health* 9, no. 1 (2013): 9–11. doi:10.2217/whe.12.69.

Chapter 9

Katz, David. "The Case for Eating 'Mostly Plants,' in 260 Words." *The Huffington Post,* April 9, 2012. http://www.huffingtonpost.com/david -katz-md/healthy-diet_b_1410803.html (accessed March 17, 2014).

U.C. San Diego Center for Integrative Medicine. "How Acupuncture Can Relieve Pain and Improve Sleep, Digestion and Emotional Well-Being." http://cim.ucsd.edu/clinical-care/acupuncture.shtml (accessed March 17, 2014).

Kim, G. S., C. H. Kim, J. Y. Park, K. U. Lee, and C. S. Park. "Effects of Vitamin B12 on Cell Proliferation and Cellular Alkaline Phosphatase

Activity in Human Bone Marrow Stromal Osteoprogenitor Cells and UMR106 Osteoblastic Cells." *Metabolism* 45, no. 12 (1996): 1443–46. doi:10.1016/S0026-0495(96)90171-7.

Dhonukshe-Rutten, R. A., S. M. Pluijm, L. C. De Groot, P. Lips, J. H. Smit, and W. A. Van Staveren. "Homocysteine and Vitamin B12 Status Relate to Bone Turnover Markers, Broadband Ultrasound Attenuation, and Fractures in Healthy Elderly People." *Journal of Bone and Mineral Research* 20, no. 6 (2005): 921–29. doi:10.1359/JBMR.050202.

Sanaka, M., T. Yamamoto, and Y. Kuyama. "Effects of Proton Pump Inhibitors on Gastric Emptying: A Systematic Review." *Digestive Diseases and Sciences* 55, no. 9 (2010): 2431–40. doi:10.1007/s10620-009-1076-x.

Pollan, Michael. *In Defense of Food: An Eater's Manifesto.* New York: Penguin Press, 2008.

Yu, Z. S., Y. C. Yu, and S. T. Sun. "The Effect of Acupuncture at Zusanli with Different Twirling Strengths on Small Intestinal Motility in Rabbits." *Chinese Acupuncture* 1 (1981): 34–37.

Zhou L, L. G. Liu, H. L. Chen, W. Y. Zhou, Y. F. Li, and M. H. Shi. "The Effect of Acupuncture 'Renzhong' on Gastric Motility and Its Relation to Peripheral 5-Hydroxytryptamine [article in Chinese]." *Zhen Ci Yan Jiu [Acupuncture Research]* 12, no. 2 (1987): 130–38.

Chapter 10

Sellmeyer, D. E., K. L. Stone, A. Sebastian, and S. R. Cummings. "A High Ratio of Dietary Animal to Vegetable Protein Increases the Rate of Bone Loss and the Risk of Fracture in Postmenopausal Women." *American Journal of Clinical Nutrition* 73, no. 1 (2001): 118–22. http://www.ncbi.nlm.nih.gov/pubmed/11124760 (accessed March 17, 2014).

Olendzki, B. C., T. D. Silverstein, G. M. Persuitte, Y. Ma, K. R. Baldwin, and D. Cave. "An Anti-Inflammatory Diet as Treatment for Inflammatory Bowel Disease: A Case Series Report." *Nutrition Journal* 13, no. 1 (2014): 5. doi:10.1186/1475-2891-13-5.

Miura, Y., H. Kato, and T. Noguchi. "Effect of Dietary Proteins on Insulin-Like Growth Factor-1 (IGF-1) Messenger Ribonucleic Acid Content in Rat Liver." *British Journal of Nutrition* 67, no. 02 (1992): 257–65. doi:10.1079/BJN19920029.

Weiss, L. A., E. Barrett-Connor, and D. Von Mühlen. "Ratio of N-6 to

N-3 Fatty Acids and Bone Mineral Density in Older Adults: The Rancho Bernardo Study." *American Journal of Clinical Nutrition* 81, no. 4 (2005): 934–38. http://www.ncbi.nlm.nih.gov/pubmed/?term=Ratio+of +N-6+to+N-3+Fatty+Acids+and+Bone+Mineral+Density+in+Older +Adults%3A+The+Rancho+Bernardo+Study (accessed April 9, 2014).

Naghii, M. R., P. Darvishi, Y. Ebrahimpour, G. Ghanizadeh, M. Mofid, M. Hedayati, and A. R. Asgari. "Effect of Combination Therapy of Fatty Acids, Calcium, Vitamin D and Boron with Regular Physical Activity on Cardiovascular Risk Factors in Rat." *Journal of Oleo Science* 61, no. 2 (2012): 103–11. doi:10.5650/jos.61.103.

Mundy, Gregory R. "Osteoporosis and Inflammation." *Nutrition Reviews* 65 (2007): S147–51. doi:10.1111/j.1753-4887.2007.tb00353.x.

Berger Ritchie, J. A., and S. L. Gerstenberger. "An Evaluation of Lead Concentrations in Imported Hot Sauces." *Journal of Environmental Science and Health, Part B* 48, no. 7 (2013): 530–38. doi:10.1080/03601234 .2013.774226.

Campbell, J. R., and M. P. Estey. "Metal Release from Hip Prostheses: Cobalt and Chromium Toxicity and the Role of the Clinical Laboratory." *Clinical Chemistry and Laboratory Medicine* 51, no. 1 (2013): 213–20. doi:10.1515/cclm-2012-0492.

Harinarayan, C. V., T. Ramalakshmi, U. V. Prasad, D. Sudhakar, P. V. Srinivasarao, K. V. Sarma, and E. G. Kumar. "High Prevalence of Low Dietary Calcium, High Phytate Consumption, and Vitamin D Deficiency in Healthy South Indians." *American Journal of Clinical Nutrition* 85, no. 4 (2007): 1062–67. http://www.ncbi.nlm.nih.gov/pubmed/?term =High+Prevalence+of+Low+Dietary+Calcium%2C+High+Phytate +Consumption%2C+and+Vitamin+D+Deficiency+in+Healthy+South +Indians (accessed April 9, 2014).

Harvard School of Public Health. "Calcium and Milk." http://www.hsph .harvard.edu/nutritionsource/what-should-you-eat/calcium-and-milk (accessed March 17, 2014).

Waring, R. H. "Report on Absorption of Magnesium Sulfate (Epsom Salts) Across the Skin." http://www.mgwater.com/transdermal.shtml (accessed March 18, 2014).

Simpson, Lani. "Vitamin D Winter." http://www.lanisimpson.com/2013 /01/25/vitamin-d-winter-2/#sthash.3AZUNqlS.dpuf (accessed March 18, 2014).

Jehle, S., H. N. Hulter, and R. Krapf. "Effect of Potassium Citrate on Bone Density, Microarchitecture, and Fracture Risk in Healthy Older Adults Without Osteoporosis: A Randomized Controlled Trial." *Journal of Clinical Endocrinology & Metabolism* 98, no. 1 (2013): 207–17. doi:10.1210 /jc.2012-3099.

Bruso, Jessica. "Which Foods Is Silicon Found In?" Last modified February 28, 2014. http://www.livestrong.com/article/170903-what-food-is -silicon-found-in/#ixzz2fme4J94i (accessed April 9, 2014).

ADAM, Inc. "Phosphorus." Last modified May 7, 2013. http://umm.edu /health/medical/altmed/supplement/phosphorus (accessed April 9, 2014).

Okyay, E., C. Ertugrul, B. Acar, A. R. Sisman, B. Onvural, and D. Ozaksoy. "Comparative Evaluation of Serum Levels of Main Minerals and Postmenopausal Osteoporosis." *Maturitas* 76, no. 4 (2013): 320–25. doi :10.1016/j.maturitas.2013.07.015.

Seo, H., Y. Cho, T. Kim, H. Shin, and I. Kwun. "Zinc May Increase Bone Formation Through Stimulating Cell Proliferation, Alkaline Phosphatase Activity and Collagen Synthesis in Osteoblastic MC3T3-El Cells." *Nutrition Research and Practice* 4, no. 5 (2010): 356–61. doi:10.4162/nrp .2010.4.5.356.

Warner, Laurie. "Copper-Zinc Imbalance: Unrecognized Consequence of Plant-Based Diets and a Contributor to Chronic Fatigue." February 14, 2008. http://www.westonaprice.org/metabolic-disorders/copper-zinc -imbalance (accessed March 18, 2014).

Iitsuka, N., M. Hie, and I. Tsukamoto. "Zinc Supplementation Inhibits the Increase in Osteoclastogenesis and Decrease in Osteoblastogenesis in Streptozotocin-induced Diabetic Rats." *European Journal of Pharmacology* 714, nos. 1–3 (2013): 41–47. doi:10.1016/j.ejphar.2013.05.020.

ADAM, Inc. "Manganese." Last modified May 7, 2013. http://umm.edu /health/medical/altmed/supplement/manganese#ixzz2fs0iPCzP (accessed April 9, 2014).

Nielsen, F. H., C. D. Hunt, L. M. Mullen, and J. R. Hunt. "Effect of Dietary Boron on Mineral, Estrogen, and Testosterone Metabolism in Postmenopausal Women." *Journal of the Federation of American Societies for Experimental Biology* 1, no. 5 (1987): 394–97. doi:10.1016/0378-5122 (88)90033-3.

Xu, P., W. B. Hu, X. Guo, Y. G. Zhang, Y. F. Li, J. F. Yao, and Q. K. Cai. "Therapeutic Effect of Dietary Boron Supplement on Retinoic Acid-Induced Osteoporosis in Rats [article in Chinese]." *Nan Fang Yi Ke Da Xue Xue Bao [Journal of Southern Medical University]* 26, no. 12 (2006): 1785–88. http://www.ncbi.nlm.nih.gov/pubmed/17259120 (accessed April 9, 2014).

Pathak, Dipali. "Vitamin C Protects, Maintains Healthy Bone Mass." *Baylor College of Medicine News,* May 11, 2010. https://www.bcm.edu/news/bones-joints-and-muscles/vitamin-c-protects-maintains-healthy-bones (accessed March 18, 2014).

Herrmann, W., S. H. Kirsch, V. Kruse, R. Eckert, S. Gräber, J. Geisel, and R. Obeid. "One Year B and D Vitamins Supplementation Improves Metabolic Bone Markers." *Clinical Chemistry and Laboratory Medicine* 51, no. 3 (2013): 639–47. doi:10.1515/cclm-2012-0599.

Keser, I., J. Z. Ilich, N. Vrkić, Z. Giljević, and I. Colić Barić. "Folic Acid and Vitamin B12 Supplementation Lowers Plasma Homocysteine but Has No Effect on Serum Bone Turnover Markers in Elderly Women: A Randomized, Double-Blind, Placebo-Controlled Trial." *Nutrition Research* 33, no. 3 (2013): 211–19. doi:10.1016/j.nutres.2013.01.002.

El Maghraoui, A., I. Ghozlani, A. Mounach, A. Rezqi, K. Oumghar, L. Achemlal, A. Bezza, and Z. Ouzzif. "Homocysteine, Folate, and Vitamin B12 Levels and Vertebral Fracture Risk in Postmenopausal Women." *Journal of Clinical Densitometry* 15, no. 3 (2012): 328–33. doi:10.1016/j.jocd.2011.12.001.

Gommans, J., Q. Yi, J. W. Eikelboom, G. J. Hankey, C. Chen, and H. Rodgers. "The Effect of Homocysteine-Lowering with B-Vitamins on Osteoporotic Fractures in Patients with Cerebrovascular Disease: Substudy of VITATOPS, a Randomised Placebo-Controlled Trial." *BMC Geriatrics* 13, no. 1 (2013): 88. doi:10.1186/1471-2318-13-88.

Sato, Y., K. Ouchi, Y. Funase, K. Yamauchi, and T. Aizawa. "Relationship Between Metformin Use, Vitamin B12 Deficiency, Hyperhomocysteinemia and Vascular Complications in Patients with Type 2 Diabetes." *Endocrine Journal* 60, no. 12 (2013): 1275–80. doi:10.1507/endocrj.EJ13-0332.

Thomas, D. "The Mineral Depletion of Foods Available to Us as a Nation (1940–2002): A Review of the 6th Edition of McCance and Widdowson." *Nutrition and Health* 19, nos. 1–2 (2007): 21–55. doi:10.1177/026010600701900205.

LiveScience Staff. "Human Gut Loaded with More Bacteria Than Thought." November 18, 2008. http://www.livescience.com/3092-human -gut-loaded-bacteria-thought.html (accessed March 18, 2014).

Doheny, Kathleen. "Anti-Inflammatory Diet: Road to Good Health?" http://www.webmd.com/food-recipes/features/anti-inflammatory-diet -road-to-good-health (accessed April 5, 2014).

National Institutes of Health. "Calcium: Dietary Supplement Fact Sheet." http://ods.od.nih.gov/factsheets/Calcium-HealthProfessional (accessed April 5, 2014).

Saito, M. "Nutrition and Bone Health. Roles of Vitamin C and Vitamin B as Regulators of Bone Mass and Quality [article in Japanese]." *Clinical Calcium* 19, no. 8 (2009): 1192–99. doi:CliCa090811921199.

Shealy, C. Norman. "Transdermal Absorption of Magnesium." *Southern Medical Journal* 98, no. 10 (2005): S18. doi:10.1097/00007611-200510001 -00038.

Rhéaume-Bleue, Kate. *Vitamin K2 and the Calcium Paradox: How a Little-Known Vitamin Could Save Your Life.* Mississauga, Ont.: J. Wiley & Sons Canada, 2012.

Davis, William. "Protecting Bone and Arterial Health with Vitamin K2." *Life Extension Magazine,* March 2008. http://www.lef.org/magazine /mag2008/mar2008_Protecting-Bone-And-Arterial-Health-With -Vitamin-K2_01.htm (accessed April 9, 2014).

Dean, Carolyn. "Magnesium Is Crucial for Bones." *The Huffington Post,* June 15, 2012. http://www.huffingtonpost.com/carolyn-dean-md-nd /bone-health_b_1540931.html (accessed March 18, 2014).

Chapter 11

Pratelli, E., I. Cinotti, and P. Pasquetti. "Rehabilitation in Osteoporotic Vertebral Fractures." *Clinical Cases in Mineral and Bone Metabolism* 7, no. 1 (2010): 45–47. http://www.ncbi.nlm.nih.gov/pmc/articles/PMC 2898006 (accessed March 18, 2014).

American Academy of Orthopaedic Surgeons. "Hip Fracture Preven-tion." http://orthoinfo.aaos.org/topic.cfm?topic=A00309 (accessed May 16, 2014).

Rector, R. S., R. Rogers, M. Ruebel, M. O. Widzer, and P. S. Hinton. "Lean Body Mass and Weight-Bearing Activity in the Prediction of

Bone Mineral Density in Physically Active Men." *Journal of Strength and Conditioning Research* 23, no. 2 (2009): 427–35. http://www.ncbi .nlm.nih.gov/pubmed/19197207 (accessed May 16, 2014). doi:10.1519/JSC .0b013e31819420e1.

National Osteoporosis Foundation. "Exercise for Strong Bones." http:// nof.org/articles/238 (accessed April 5, 2014).

Iwamoto, J., T. Takeda, and Y. Sato. "Interventions to Prevent Bone Loss in Astronauts During Space Flight." *The Keio Journal of Medicine* 54, no. 2 (2005): 55–59. doi:10.2302/kjm.54.55.

Sibonga, J. D., H. J. Evans, H. G. Sung, F. R. Spector, T. F. Lang, V. S. Oganov, A. V. Bakulin, L. C. Shackelford, and A. D. Leblanc. "Recovery of Spaceflight-Induced Bone Loss: Bone Mineral Density after Long-Duration Missions as Fitted with an Exponential Function." *Bone* 41, no. 6 (2007): 973–78. doi:10.1016/j.bone.2007.08.022.

National Aeronautics and Space Administration. "Space Bones." *Science @NASA*, October 1, 2001. http://science.nasa.gov/science-news/science -at-nasa/2001/ast01oct_1 (accessed April 4, 2014).

Leung, D. P., C. K. Chan, H. W. Tsang, W. W. Tsang, and A. Y. Jones. "Tai Chi as an Intervention to Improve Balance and Reduce Falls in Older Adults: A Systematic and Meta-Analytical Review." *Alternative Therapies in Health and Medicine* 17, no. 1 (2011): 40–48. http://www.ncbi.nlm.nih .gov/pubmed/21614943 (accessed April 9, 2014).

Rubin, C., A. S. Turner, S. Bain, C. Mallinckrodt, and K. McLeod. "Anabolism: Low Mechanical Signals Strengthen Long Bones." *Nature* 412 (2001): 603–604. Doi:doi:10.1038/35088122.

Rubin, C., G. Xu, and S. Judex. "The Anabolic Activity of Bone Tissue, Suppressed by Disuse, Is Normalized by Brief Exposure to Extremely Low-Magnitude Mechanical Stimuli." *The FASEB Journal* 15, no. 12 (2001): 2225–29. Doi:10.1096/fj.01-0166com.

Judex, S., N. Zhong, M. E. Squire, K. Ye, L. Donahue, M. Hadjiargyrou, and C. T. Rubin. "Mechanical Modulation of Molecular Signals Which Regulate Anabolic and Catabolic Activity in Bone Tissue." *Journal of Cellular Biochemistry* 94, no. 5 (2005): 982–94. doi:10.1002/jcb.20363.

Kiiski, J., A. Heinonen, T. L. Järvinen, P. Kannus, and H. Sievänen. "Transmission of Vertical Whole Body Vibration to the Human

Body." *Journal of Bone and Mineral Research* 23, no. 8 (2008): 1318–25. doi:10.1359/jbmr.080315.

Rubin, C., R. Recker, D. Cullen, J. Ryaby, J. Mccabe, and K. Mcleod. "Prevention of Postmenopausal Bone Loss by a Low-Magnitude, High-Frequency Mechanical Stimuli: A Clinical Trial Assessing Compliance, Efficacy, and Safety." *Journal of Bone and Mineral Research* 19, no. 3 (2004): 343–51. doi:10.1359/JBMR.0301251.

National Institutes of Health. "Once Is Enough: A Guide to Preventing Future Fractures." January 2012. http://www.niams.nih.gov/Health_Info /bone/Osteoporosis/Fracture/default.asp (accessed April 05, 2014).

Resources

Dr. Lani Simpson's Website: www.LaniSimpson.com

CDs, DVDs, e-books, audio files, articles, webinars, recipes, an osteoporosis history form, and other useful resources on topics including osteoporosis, menopause, PMS, and hypothyroidism. Also includes two items mentioned in the book: the Diet Journal and the Bristol Stool Chart (www .LaniSimpson.com/dr-simpsons-diet-diary-and-symptom-chart).

Online Tools and Forms

American Bone Health FORE Fracture Risk Calculator: www.american bonehealth.org/tools-and-resources/risk-calculator

FRAX WHO Fracture Risk Assessment Tool: www.shef.ac.uk/FRAX /tool.jsp

My Family Health Portrait (U.S. Surgeon General): https://familyhistory .hhs.gov/fhh-web/home.action

Informational Websites

About.com Thyroid Disease: http://thyroid.about.com

BMI (body mass index) calculator: www.webmd.com/diet/calc-bmi-plus

Celiac disease: www.celiac.com

Centers for Disease Control and Prevention: www.cdc.gov

Christiane Northrup, MD: www.drnorthrup.com

Environmental Working Group: www.EWG.org

Foundation for Osteoporosis Research (FORE): www.FORE.org

International Osteoporosis Foundation (IOF): www.iofbonehealth.org

International Society of Clinical Densitometry (ISCD): www.ISCD.org

Irma Jennings (Food for Healthy Bones): www.foodforhealthybones.com

National Association of Nutrition Professionals (NANP): www.nanp.org

National Bone Health Alliance: www.2million2many.org

National Institutes of Health: www.niams.nih.gov/Health_Info/Bone
/Osteoporosis/Fracture/default.asp#b

National Osteoporosis Foundation: http://nof.org

Natural Resources Defense Council (NRDC): www.nrdc.org

North American Menopause Society (information about the KEEPS
Trial): www.menopause.org

Susan Brown, PhD: www.betterbones.com

Specialty Lab Testing

BioHealth Laboratory: http://biohealthlab.com

Canary Club: www.canaryclub.org

Diagnos-Techs: www.diagnostechs.com

Genova Diagnostics: www.gdx.net

Lab Tests Online: www.labtestsonline.com (A nonprofit site where you
can look up lab tests to find out what the results mean.)

Metametrix Clinical Laboratory: www.metametrix.com

Professional Co-Op Laboratory Testing: www.professionalco-op.com
(By joining this physician's co-op of four thousand members, doctors
can receive very low prices for their patients' lab work. The doctor pays
the invoice and bills the patient. I use this service for patients who do not
have insurance. The cost is often 50 percent less than if a doctor were to
bill insurance or a patient were to pay cash. Let your doctor know about
this cost-effective way to order tests. The blood tests are drawn at any
Labcorp facility.)

ZRT Laboratory: www.zrtlab.com

Exercise and Vibration Equipment

Bellicon Rebounder: www.bellicon-usa.com

Foot Levelers and Thera-ciser exercise bands: www.footlevelers.com
/products/rehab-tools/theraciser

Jump Sport Trampolines (Rebounder): www.jumpsport.com

Juvent Dynamic Motion Therapy (Low-Intensity Vibration): http://
juventhealth.com

Marodyne Medical (Low-Intensity Vibration): www.marodyne.com

Supplement Companies

Advanced Orthomolecular Research: www.aor.ca

Biotics Research: www.bioticsresearch.com

Designs for Health: www.designsforhealth.com

Douglas Laboratory: www.douglaslabs.com

Metagenics: www.metagenics.com

Nordic Naturals: www.nordicnaturals.com

OsteoNaturals: www.osteonaturals.com

Pure Encapsulations: www.pureencapsulations.com

Standard Process: www.standardprocess.com

Thorne Research: www.thorne.com

Books

Black, Jessica K. *The Anti-Inflammation Diet and Recipe Book.* Alameda, CA: Hunter House, 2006.

Black, Jessica K. *More Anti-Inflammation Diet Tips and Recipes.* Alameda, CA: Hunter House, 2013.

Brown, Susan E. *Better Bones, Better Body: Beyond Estrogen and Calcium,* 2nd edition. New York: McGraw-Hill, 2000.

Dean, Carolyn. *The Magnesium Miracle* (revised edition). New York: Ballantine Books, 2006.

McCormick, Keith. *The Whole-Body Approach to Osteoporosis.* Oakland, CA: New Harbinger Publications, 2009.

Northrup, Christiane. *The Wisdom of Menopause: Creating Physical and Emotional Health During the Change* (revised edition). New York: Bantam, 2012.

Rhéaume-Bleue, Kate. *Vitamin K2 and the Calcium Paradox: How a Little-Known Vitamin Could Save Your Life.* New York: Harper, 2013.

Schneider, Diane L. *The Complete Book of Bone Health.* Amherst, NY: Prometheus Books, 2011.

Shames, Richard, Karilee Shames, and Georjana Grace Shames. *Thyroid Mind Power: The Proven Cure for Hormone-Related Depression, Anxiety, and Memory Loss.* New York: Rodale Books, 2011.

Shomon, Mary J. *The Thyroid Diet Revolution: Manage Your Master Gland of Metabolism for Lasting Weight Loss.* New York: William Morrow Paperbacks, 2012.

Smith, Pamela Wartian. *What You Must Know about Women's Hormones: Your Guide to Natural Hormone Treatments for PMS, Menopause, Osteoporosis, PCOS, and More.* Garden City Park, NY: Square One Publishers, 2008.

Bone Density Testing Machine Companies

General Electric: www3.gehealthcare.com/en/Products/Categories/Bone_Health

Hologic: www.hologic.com

Norland: www.coopersurgical.com/ourproducts/Pages/NorlandXR-600.aspx?name=Norland%20XR-600

Index

interest," 46; ethnic and racial differences, 59; failure to establish "least significant change" data, 45–46; false negatives, 53; false positives, 52–53; health insurance coverage of, 72–73; inaccurate selection of vertebrae, 49–50; and lack of training, 37–38; manufacturers of machines, 283; peripheral machine tests, 79–80; physicians' assessment of, 37; positioning errors, 35–37, 46; in pregnancy, 77; and previous lumbar surgeries, 70–71; reporting errors, 2, 43; retesting, 74–75, 82; rushed testing, 44; and scoliosis, 70–71; site discordance, 53, 79–80; in small-boned people, 52–53; standard deviations, 58; technologists' training, 37, 40; test anxiety, 77; vertebral fracture assessment (VFA), 80–81. *See also* DXA (dual-energy X-ray absorptiometry)
Bone Health and Osteoporosis, 42–43
bone loss: active, 112; age-related, 9–10; and hypothyroidism, 183–184; in men, 9
bone marker tests, 118–119
bone marrow fat, 10
bone mass, 14
bone mineral density (BMD), 5, 13–14, 57
bone remodeling, 11–13, 128–129
bone scan, 65–66
bone strength versus density, 15, 246
bones, growth process of, 8–13
Boniva, 126, 129, 130, 142
boron, recommended amount, 253
bowel movements, and digestive health, 204–209
Brenner, Judith, 87–88
Bristol Stool Chart, 208

C
calcitonin, 148–149, 173, 174, 183
calcitriol, 119, 173, 174–175
calcium: coral, 163; and heart disease, 245–246; overdosing on, 244–245; products for bone-building, 163–164; raw, 163–164; recommended amounts, 28, 242–246; tests, 115–116
Camacho, Pauline, 141

candida yeast, 217
carbohydrates, recommended amounts, 233–234
CBC (complete blood count) test, 114
celiac disease, 117, 186, 210–211, 223
celiac profile test, 117
Cenestin, 191
Centers for Disease Control, 29, 31
certified bone densitometry technologist (CBDT), 38–39
certified clinical densitometrist (CCD), 39
chamomile, 225
children and bone health, 28–29
Chinese herbal supplements, 157–158
chiropractic, 166–167
Chopra, Deepak, 153
Cleveland Clinic Journal of Medicine, 139
Clinical Rheumatology, 46
Clinician's Guide to Prevention and Treatment of Osteoporosis, 134
colon, 201–203, 216
complementary treatment, 154
comprehensive blood chemistry panel, 114
constipation, 205–206, 228
copper, recommended amount, 253
coral calcium, 163
core training, 267
cortisol, 107–108, 117–118, 182
cortisone, 97
creatinine test, 116
Crohn's disease, 216
Cushing's disease, 117

D
dandelion root, 226
Dean, Carolyn, 247
degenerative joint disease (DJD), 27
dehydration, 228, 234–235
denosumab (Prolia), 145–146
densitometry: certification in, 37, 75–76; lack of professional training, 2; overview of, 38–41
DHEA, 181, 192
diarrhea, 206–207
Didronel, 129, 130
diet: carbohydrates, recommended amounts, 234–235; elimination, 222–223; fats, recommended